THE RELENTLESS
PURSUIT OF PEACE

The Relentless Pursuit of Peace

A Roadmap to Mental Health

Max Coates

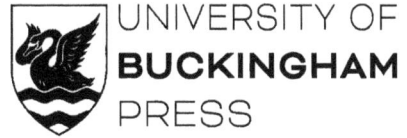

UNIVERSITY OF BUCKINGHAM PRESS,
AN IMPRINT OF LEGEND TIMES GROUP LTD
51 Gower Street
London WC1E 6HJ
United Kingdom
www.unibuckinghampress.com

First published by University of Buckingham Press in 2024

© Max Coates, 2024

The right of the author to be identified as the author of this work has been asserted in accordance with the Copyright, Designs and Patents Act 1988. British Library Cataloguing in Publication Data available.

ISBN: 9781917163828

All rights reserved. No part of this publication may be reproduced, stored in or introduced into a retrieval system, or transmitted, in any form or by any means (electronic, mechanical, photocopying, recording or otherwise), without the prior written permission of the publisher. This book is sold subject to the condition that it shall not be resold, lent, hired out or otherwise circulated without the express prior consent of the publisher.

CONTENTS

Foreword — vii

Introduction — 3

1. It's complicated (or is it?) — 11
2. It's doing my head in — 25
3. A perfect storm — 35
4. Did I mention stress? — 46
5. Too much, too far, too soon or too long — 58
6. Upcycle — 73
7. How low can you get? — 84
8. Living the Dream — 96
9. Breaking bad — 105
10. Great expectations — 112
11. Hall of mirrors — 121
12. Strategic Selfishness — 136
13. The Blind Woodturner — 145
14. Strike a happy media — 154
15. Simples — 166
16. Toast — 172
17. Zen and the art of spoon carving — 181
18. The relentless pursuit of peace — 192

References — 204

Foreword

I have known the author Max, for around 15 years. We first met at University College London when I was invited to speak to one of his groups of Masters' students on the topic of 'coaching and beyond'. We hit it off straight away, and that he was not offended by my remarking how much he resembled Tom Baker's Dr Who, is a testament to the very rich and dear friendship that has grown out of our various professional collaborations and personal challenges over this past decade and a half.

I have felt immensely privileged to read chapters of this book as it has been written, rewritten, thrown out and begun again. Your next book Max is to be called "The Resilient Writer". I know Max, at times, it has been like birthing a fully-spined echidna for you. But you have persevered and here it is, in all its glory. Even if you've also laid an egg writing it.

I have been able to admire the genius that operates between his ears when spinning his narrative silk, and witnessed a man wanting to delight, challenge and inspire his readers, with a burning passion to make the world a better place.

This book brings together a rich neuroscientific, psychological and social history of the mind. Expertly casting and weaving an enchanting web within which to wrap tasty morsels of tantalising facts and statistics. Do you know for example how many thousands of parts an average car is made of? Or what the weight of an ostrich is in chicken nugget form? Max takes the reader on an emotional roller coaster, exploring the very serious business of the state of our mental health in modern society, how and why it faulters, and the very tangible things we can do to raise that state to something approaching vitality.

Max draws on his own rich experience as an educator, academic, counsellor and priest to spin a thoroughly evidenced narrative that argues for change. It argues for shift at a corporate, organisational and societal level. At the same time presents that rare quality of offering a real, practical and essential guide to better mental health for us as individuals; grounded in the reality of our daily lives.

His trademark humour will have you laughing out loud, and his erudite command of the academic and clinical literature around old and new models of brain function, polyvagal theory and modern theories of trauma recovery, will open your eyes to the new dawn of emotional health and well-being that awaits us.

In addition to charting the development of neurological and psychological knowledge from the literature, Max also presents his own synthesis in the form of his ground-breaking new model of emotional and mental well-being. His 'Structure of Mental Health Model' neatly brings together all the threads of his arguments into one succinct and visually striking framework. A kind of audit of audacious well-being.

Max pushes at the edge of so many 'accepted' norms around depression and anxiety and the medicalisation of 'dis-eases' of the psyche. He eruditely challenges the 'pharmaceuticalisation' of mental health, using clinical research (not conspiracy theory!). Questioning the efficacy and modality of anti-depressants and their dubious use in the under 24's, based on their well -documented and horrifying side effects.

I am particularly excited by his ground-breaking inclusion of Emotional Freedom Techniques (EFT) in his book. EFT, once side-lined as an 'energy therapy' and daubed with a 'Woowoo' bumper sticker, has become a force majeure in the treatment of PTSD and Complex PTSD, burnout, depression, pain management and anxiety. Boasting over 1500 research papers many coming from the prestigious Peta Stapleton and Dawson Church camp of the Antipodes, EFT is a cutting-edge therapy with real promise. It sits in the Sensorimotor Pyschotherapies branch of trauma treatment and has attracted the attention of the UK's National Institute for Clinical Excellence (NICE). Max gives EFT centre stage and also explains how you, the reader, can use this simple and effective approach to manage unhelpful thoughts and feelings.

Finally, I know Max so well, and I know he is no stranger to personal adversity. He hides it well, but his struggles with his health have given ample opportunity to prove that what he writes about, is also what he lives. He practices his preachings, and it is a testament to him that he is still writing and researching with such vigour, rigor and energy. And as always with such devout integrity for the pursuit of truth in the service of others.

If you want a book that is a dry and stuffy academic assessment of the state of mental health and how to improve it, you won't find it here. Or at least you will find it, in a rigorously evidenced and beautifully constructed narrative. You will also find a rich and fascinating psychosocial history and both poignant and very humorous anecdotes that bring mental health to the fore, and challenge you to think out of the box and out of the page.

Prepare to be entertained, and to be surprised. Prepare to be challenged, and be prepared to change your mind. Is that not what a good book should do for the reader?

Thank you for writing this book Max, I know it has been

immensely challenging on so many levels, but my goodness the world needs this, and it needs it right now.

Will Thomas MA., BSc(Hons), PGCE
Coach, EFT Practitioner, Hypnotherapist and Fellow Spoon Carver

THE RELENTLESS PURSUIT OF PEACE

Introduction

There was a time when talking about personal mental health issues was seen as being tantamount to a public confession of inadequacy. My maternal grandmother suffered with her nerves, my youth leader committed suicide and a colleague in my first job was often absent as part of the legacy of the inhumane treatment he suffered as a prisoner of war. These people and many others that I have met were distressed but were often discussed in hushed tones or even worse not discussed at all. Perhaps, those around them were dealing with their own concerns and even their fears when faced with such unfathomable behaviours.

Times have changed and it is increasingly acceptable to talk about personal mental health issues. Surely, this is a positive shift and will help level the playing field between the acceptability of discussing physical and mental illnesses? Sometimes such discussions about the latter could have veered too far and moved from being informative and even therapeutic towards a little too much personal introspection and even teetering on the edge of being self-indulgent.

More recently the Covid 19 Pandemic gripped our attention in 2020 and has led to unexpected changes in our life experiences. My own observations suggest that there is a residual anxiety and even a social reticence as Covid has hopefully subsided. There has been an additional overlay with Putin's war in Ukraine. Events like these certainly turn up the volume on mental health.

Social media has frequently become a driver for developing and extending mental health issues. People share intimate thoughts and concerns and bring them into an all too public domain. The response to their candour is not always constructive. At the time of writing, the inquest into the tragic suicide in 2017 of teenager Molly Russell has just been concluded. The BBC reported the following comments by her father, Ian: 'It's time to protect our innocent young people instead of allowing [social media] platforms to prioritise their profits by monetising the misery of children. (Crawford and Bell 2022).

There have always been people whose mental health can crumble to a destructive and distressing extent. However, whether as a result of increased diagnosis, circumstances or discussion, there has been a sharp rise in the incidence of people struggling in this way. I was talking to a friend who had been to an appointment with their beauty therapist. The beautician described a conversation with her two teenage daughters. They were offering their mother a catalogue of their friends' mental health issues: anxiety, depression, ADHD, separation anxiety etc. The girls asked their mother what her friends suffered with. The mother replied 'Not a lot', a response which astonished her daughters. Could it be that we are too ready to provide labels rather than tools for coping with the consequences of living in our overstretched, media-obsessed lives? Perhaps, we have not been adequately prepared for the disappointments and problems that life can bring with its inevitable tidal flow of personal highs and lows. The intention of this book is not about creating another diagnostic manual to pigeonhole mental health issues. The book does not provide an alternative panacea for individuals receiving clinical support for distressing and debilitating mental conditions. Rather, this is an open letter to the many, who like me, have hit more bumps in the road than expected. It is targeted at keeping our thoughts, dreams and emotional health in a better place.

A sea change in my own thinking came in my late twenties when I was trained as a counsellor by Anthony Clare (later the presenter of *In the Psychiatrist's Chair* on Radio 4). At the time that I met him, Dr Clare was an embryonic firebrand at the Royal Maudsley and Bethlem Hospital in London. His influence opened my eyes to the impact of life events and the allied stress and the centrality of working to secure significant change in an individual's achievement, behaviour and stability. Before studying with him, my view was that if people enjoyed different circumstances and opportunities then they would flourish. I had been committed to structural reform within society, in my case through my work in education. Nobody wants to see widespread poverty and restricted opportunities. However, Dr Clare made me aware of the complexity that surrounds motivation, mental health and behaviour. He started me on a journey that has both fascinated and perplexed. This book is about my progress to date.

The majority of my professional life has been spent in education; in schools as a secondary school science teacher, then as a school leader and finally as a university academic with University College London (UCL). My career did not turn out as I expected but there was always the constant of working with people. In my career I have been threatened by crazed parents, even to the point of having a gun fired at me. I have had to respond to significant safeguarding issues. I saw colleagues burn out, break down and even be arrested. I recall the intense sadness of finding out that a teacher colleague had thrown themselves off a motorway bridge leaving a preschool age family behind. In 2005 terrorists blew up a bus in Tavistock Square in London. This was near to where I was working at UCL. Thirteen innocent people lost their lives. The explosion rattled our office windows and many of us were left unsettled and anxious in the following weeks and months.

In every situation that I have worked in I saw the same repeated behaviours as people tried to cope with the pressures and circumstances of living and working. Most struggled with stress resulting from the pressure of work, redundancy, financial worries, sleep deprivation caused by their young families, divorce, bereavement, illness, past events staging a reprise in their current thinking, train strikes, climate change, toxic relationships and a cacophony of other intrusions. Of course, stress does not come from difficult times, even good times can cause it. Just think of making the move to the house of your dreams or the birth of a child.

In 2003 I was faced with a dilemma. I was working with senior staff in organisations around developing vision, teams and restructuring and training in a form of coaching which was limited to goal setting and decision making. I was routinely faced with these same people who were highly stressed even to the point of becoming professionally and personally dysfunctional. My choice was to concentrate on the pragmatic organisational concerns and leave the issues around personal function to take their course; to be honest, a much easier option. Two events in a single week helped me resolve that dilemma. I was working with a CEO who was merging two organisations, textbook planning or so I had assumed. However, she suddenly confided with me that every time she had to speak to a group of people, she was physically sick. Could I help, because she found the problem so embarrassing that resigning was under serious consideration?

The second encounter was with the principal of a large London comprehensive school. His was a challenging role at the best of times. Significant changes in government policy allied to operating with a toxic leadership team had raised his stress levels. Such was the intensity of this stress that he was dissociating and could only talk about himself in the third person. Trivial? I can only remember the encounter as being very disconcerting.

I decided at the end of that week to try to find ways of supporting people: those individuals that I was encountering, personally and professionally, people whose expectations had been shattered and who were carrying a load beyond their personal capacity. I recommenced that fascinating journey which had started some years ago with Anthony Clare and which is the basis of this book.

Almost immediately, I discovered that there was a great deal of misleading information around brain function and mental health much of which was being circulated as fact. For example, many people were undergoing psychometric tests which sought to define them and which had extremely limited substance. These were, and indeed still are, being used to make appointments and steer career paths within organisations. They have the potential to leave a legacy of distorted personal identity and impose a mental straight jacket. At the time, a management consultant told me that some mutual friends were getting divorced. He is a dedicated Myers-Briggs Type Indicator (MBTI) practitioner. He followed up his news by telling me that they should never have got married in the first place because their MBTI four letter designations were not aligned. His unsupported views were certainly closer to astrology than psychology by a country mile.

Management consultants and trainers have persistently used a model of the brain that understands the evolution of our brains as a series of overlays. This model originated with Paul MacLean in the 1960s but detailed in a later publication in 1990. Labelled the 'Triune Brain', it identifies the lowest part as reptilian, then the next overlay is the limbic centre, then as a final tour de force, the seat of thinking and rationality, the neocortex. His model depicts a battlefield with rational thinking seeking to hold emotion in check. This model is persistent and routinely used in leadership and management training sessions. The influential psycho journalist, Daniel Goleman, drew heavily on it and shaped a generation of leadership and educational thinking. Using MacLean's model he tried to recast the contribution of the middle layer, the limbic system, in constructive terms.

> The ultimate act of personal responsibility at work may be in taking control of our own state of mind. Moods exert a powerful pull on thought, memory and perception. When we are angry, we more readily remember incidents that support our ire, our thoughts become preoccupied with the object of our anger, irritability so skews our worldview that an otherwise benign comment might now strike us as hostile. Resisting this despotic quality of moods is essential to our ability to work productively. (Goleman, 1998, p. 83)

There are some parts of that quotation which might even sit reasonably with the arguments of this book. However, a giveaway around his thinking is that he uses a phrase such as 'despotic quality' and postulates the limbic centre as being a threat to our effective performance. Writers such as Goleman treat this emotion-generating part of the brain with a degree of suspicion and even fear. In Charlotte Brontë's 1847 novel,

Jane Eyre, Mr Rochester's insane and unpredictable first wife is kept locked in the attic under supervision of a nurse. Eventually, Bertha escapes, with dire consequences. I find it difficult to read Goleman without *Jane Eyre* running in parallel. Our limbic centre, even if we had one, is not the mad relative in the attic.

Those still using this model portray the inner workings of the brain as being locked in a battle trying to favour rationality over emotion. There is, however, a flaw in MacLean's model and in all the cover versions that have followed on for over 70 years. It is quite simply wrong. Our brains are neither structured, as he asserted, nor do they function in the manner which he predicted. More on this later in the book.

Over the last twenty years I have explored psychotherapy, Reverse Therapy, Emotional Freedom Technique (EFT), psychology, hypnotherapy, coaching, and mindfulness. My own doctorate was around emotional intelligence. I have published some of my earlier thinking – see Coates (2008) and Coates (2018). These two were very much set in an educational context. In this book I have sought to widen my audience and it is, well – about you (and me)! I will share some of my findings. My own work with individuals has evolved in this journey of exploration but pragmatism alone can never be enough and so each proffered insight is rooted in evidence and research.

Some of the most enriching experiences in my life have been conversations with friends and colleagues. My life has been like an extended railway journey with some fellow passengers joining me in my carriage for short periods and others travelling with me for the duration. Many have contributed unwittingly to what follows whilst others have been willingly complicit in its genesis. I am grateful for all the contributions, but the book's inadequacies are entirely mine.

My particular thanks go to Will Thomas for his advice and for writing the foreword and for providing a literary shoulder to cry on. I have also greatly valued my conversations with Professor Anthony Clare, John West – Burnham, Dr Domini Bingham, Dr Chris Moran, Professor Kathryn Riley, Les Symonds, Mark Tyrell, Anthony Jacquin, and Dr John Eaton. Also, Professor Ian Craig who has earthed my thinking with a healthy dose of scepticism. Thanks, also, go to my son Steve for a number of the graphics and providing IT 'roadside assistance'. Alex Sharratt, the editor at John Catt Educational, has kindly allowed me to use some of my use ideas and text drawn from an earlier book, *It's Doing My Head In* (2018).

Thanks are due to Jonathan Reuvid and Tom Chalmers and the team at my publisher, University of Buckingham Press. Their technical assistance – and indeed their belief that I could craft this book – has been greatly valued.

My wife, Sally, has sourced anecdotes and tea, her most impressive contribution has been her ability to cook supper for friends whilst listening to me read sections of this book at the least inappropriate time. We really must get out more.

1
IT'S COMPLICATED (OR IS IT?)

> How can a three-pound mass of jelly that you can hold in your palm imagine angels, contemplate the meaning of infinity, and even question its own place in the cosmos? Especially awe-inspiring is the fact that any single brain, including yours, is made up of atoms that were forged in the hearts of countless, far-flung stars billions of years ago. These particles drifted for eons and light-years until gravity and change brought them together here, now. These atoms now form a conglomerate – your brain – that can not only ponder the very stars that gave it birth but can also think about its own ability to think and wonder about its own ability to wonder. With the arrival of humans, it has been said, the universe has suddenly become conscious of itself. This, truly, is the greatest mystery of all.
> (Ramachandran, 2012, p. 7)

Our brains are incredibly complex, with each one containing around 100 billion nerve cells or neurons. This is more than the number of stars in the Milky Way. That is just the start, as each neuron can connect with perhaps 10,000 others. This allows for the possibility of some 100 trillion nerve connections. If each of these neurons was laid end-to-end, they would circle the earth twice. This incredible level of complexity challenges us not to trivialise psychology. That quote, also, captures something of our feelings of awe, as complex individuals in the context of a vast universe. It leaves us considering that we might indeed be stardust and it sets a high bar for our personal potential.

Ramachandran's rhetoric is impressive. I would also argue that it is flawed and perhaps even irresponsible. Step back a moment from the '*Mr. Fahrenheit*' imagery (Mercury 1978) and earth your thinking in experiences which are all too often grittier and certainly far less triumphalist than the Ramachandran quote. Imagine that it is February, with its characteristic dull skies; the pandemic has remained unexpectedly persistent, the cost of living is accelerating and for many expenditure is exceeding income. The relationship with your partner is tense, whilst at work there might be rumours going around about redundancies. Somehow, that contemplation of being at the edge of the universe shudders to a halt.

American psychiatrist, Peck (1978) took an altogether more realistic view when he pointed out:

Life is difficult.

This is a great truth, one of the greatest truths. It is a great truth because once we truly see this truth, we transcend it. Once we truly know that life is difficult – once we truly understand and accept it – then life is no longer difficult. Because, once it is accepted, the fact that is difficult no longer matters. when we see this truth. (p. 3)

For many of us, Peck's words connect with our daily experience. Simply accepting that the highway of life is rutted, unpredictable and full of potholes is Victim 101 and places us very much at the mercy of circumstances. However, if we are prepared to step up a level and move from resignation to the confrontation of our challenges, then we begin to generate solutions; suddenly our victimhood becomes stripped of its enervating power.

The sun may come out tomorrow. However, having an umbrella and investing in wellies could well be a prudent approach.

THE MAMMOTH IN THE ROOM

There is a danger that we can confuse cultural change with the rate of biological evolution. We are surrounded by the incredible outcomes of human ingenuity, creativity and enterprise: Michelangelo's ceiling in the Sistine Chapel, Einstein's Theory of Special Relativity or Renzo Piano's Shard of Glass building in London. From my bathroom window I can see the house where Berners-Lee, the scientist who conceptualised the World Wide Web, used to live. I routinely supervise students in: Beijing, Zurich, Chile and Kazakhstan without even leaving my home in Dorset. This acceleration in our communications, inventions, culture and social complexity must, surely, be in step with the evolutionary development of our brains?

This is not the case. Evolution simply does not move that fast. It is unlikely that our brains have undergone any significant changes for perhaps 50,000 years. Our Palaeolithic ancestors, who were hunter-gatherers, were significantly like us. The same neural processing that enabled them to hunt woolly mammoths with relatively basic weapons also enables us to innovate and run complex organisations such as factories and hospitals. It is allowing us to embed ourselves '*Matrix like*' within social media. At this point of human history, we are engaged in relentless change and innovation either as instigators or as victims. For many, even our leisure becomes phrenetical, structured through activities such as gaming, the gym, clubbing or You Tube and we build in too little downtime, space where our brains simply idle on tick-over.

Is this assumed pace just a slow-motion car crash? To date, it does not seem to be the case. Our brains are continuing to generate creative solutions to complex problems even though our context is morphing at an ever-increasing speed. Toffler, writing nearly 50 years ago in his iconic book *Future Shock*, raised this issue of us becoming overwhelmed by an explosion of knowledge and change:

> We may define future shock as the distress, both physical and psychological, that arises from an overload of the human organism's physical adaptive systems and its decision-making processes. Put more simply, future shock is the human response to over stimulation. (1970, p. 297)

His prophetic stance generated a lot of discussion but it has not served as a reflective brake. We continue to expand the use of our brains as we handle increasing complexity and an increasing immersion in an IT based knowledge economy. Despite its plasticity, our archaic neurological system has not undergone any recent upgrades. Our brains were formatted in a very different setting. They developed in a world where daily survival was the top priority. Consequently, we at our core we have inherited a legacy of responses, such as the fight-or-flight-or-freeze mechanisms. Such legacy mechanisms are inevitably very powerful because they were honed to enhance survival in the 'now' and this will tend to eclipse longer-term goals and aspirations.

In circumstances where we are under immediate threat or pressure for longer periods of time, these now behaviours, in the very act of trying to guard, guide and protect us, can have a detrimental impact by overloading our physiology and collapsing longer term perspectives. Fight-or-flight-or-freeze works well when confronted with mammoths – indeed, it is not bad with oncoming buses. These responses are less beneficial when we are under pressure from sustained and diffuse pressures. They can be decidedly counterproductive when we are faced with long-term toxic organisational politics, relationship breakdown, health problems or financial worries

A QUICK (AND LARGELY INADEQUATE) PRIMER ON THE BRAIN

The argument of this book is that we often take great pride in being rational and in demonstrating this with measured and controlled behaviour. In practice, we are an integrated forum with many parts working together to generate decisions. When stressed, we are more likely to be driven by a counter current of less accessible brain activity where rational thinking can be overridden or even overwhelmed by a perceived need to survive. Many of us believe that we think issues through in a measured manner, consider all sides of the argument and reach a decision. However, there are just so many situations, possibly most situations, where that does not happen. Imagine getting engaged and prefacing your proposal with "I have considered all the variables, looked at the financial implications, compared you with other models currently available and decided to ask you to marry me". This approach would probably result in hospitalisation. Of course, we would not use such an approach, so is it simply an exaggeration? However, consider for a moment – where we choose to live, the car that we drive, the clothes we wear and the music that we are badged by. If you still have any doubts, go to a football match where the team is close to relegation and listen to the unbridled optimism or even the fantasy world of the fans' explanations around this. Despite a great deal of effort by the HR specialists in organisations creating tools to mitigate the potential intuitive behaviours of managers, such as the use of selection matrices in making appointments, significant decisions around applicants attending job interviews are often made in the first 90 seconds.

REALLY?

As referred to in my introduction, the evolutionary biologist, MacLean (1960) proposed that our brains were layered; in the basement was a reptilian brain handling a lot of the physiological management such as our heartrate or our breathing, then a central paleo-mammalian brain (limbic centre) with a role with emotions and memory and then finally the neocortex (neo-mammalian brain) at the front of the brain, with an emphasis on rationality and creativity. Maclean's model, the Triune Brain, has been in common usage for some sixty years. When it was published it enjoyed popularist advocates such as Sagan in his book *The Dragons of Eden* (1977) and Koestler (1967). This model has been extensively used by those working in consultancy and self-help books (Bowden 2013).

So, a bit of downtime and I picked up the thriller *Fear No Evil* by James Patterson (2022). Patterson is a bestselling American writer. In this story his hero psychologist and criminologist, Alex Ross, is flying from Denver to Paris where his wife had been the victim of a terrorist attack. His anxiety is described in the following excerpt.

> We took off and my mind started to play tricks with me. It shifted to the oldest part of the brain, the limbic system, the reptilian place where fear and worry and terrible images and impossible questions dwell and fester. (p. 160-161)

Even popular fiction is not a safe haven from unsupported and ingrained thinking. Whilst we may be dismissive about it being contained in fiction the idea is still being communicated.

This view of the brain is analogous to an apartment block complete with a cortical penthouse and has been repeatedly challenged. Barrett who is amongst is among the top 1% most cited scientists in the world for her revolutionary research in psychology and neuroscience is dismissive of the MacLean's model and in turn of its persistent adherents.

> So, you don't have an inner lizard or an emotional beast-brain. There is no such thing as a limbic centre dedicated to emotions. And your misnamed neocortex is not a new part; many other vertebrates grow the same neurons that, in some animals, organise into her cerebral cortex if key stages run for long enough. Anything you read or hear that proclaims the human neocortex, cerebral cortex, or pre-frontal cortex to be the root of rationality, or says that the frontal lobe regulates so-called emotional brain areas to keep irrational behaviour in check, is simply outdated or woefully complete. The triune brain idea and its epic battle between emotion, instinct, and rationality is a modern myth. (2020, p.24).

Once she has got the bit between her teeth, she becomes even more dismissive.

The triune brain idea is one of the most successful and widespread errors in all of science. It's certainly a compelling story at times it captures how we feel in daily life. For example, when your tastebuds are tempted to buy a luscious slice of velvety chocolate cake but you declined it because, honestly, you've just finished breakfast, it's easy to believe that your impulsive inner lizard and your emotional limbic centre pushed you in a cake-ward direction, and your rational neocortex wrestled the pair into submission. But human brains don't work that way. (Barrett, 2020, p. 15-19)

Barrett (2020) goes on to suggest that our understanding of contemporary neuroscience would be helped by using the metaphor of air travel. She suggests that air travel functions because it is networked through a series of hubs. Some airports have direct flights to other airports, but not to all. Some require passengers to change planes and move from one hub to another in order to complete their journey. In the same way she suggests that your neurones are grouped around hubs and that there is interconnection between these clusters but that communication between them is not always direct. If every single neurone was connected to every other, the capacity of our brains would need to be beyond computation. In the same way that air travel would be overwhelmed by the number of planes required to service a totally connected network. This hub model hints at organisation that is both economical and efficient.

These neural hubs may well have an area of specialism, for example sight or hearing. However, these groups of neurones can change their function. Suggesting that given areas of the brain 'light up' in response to a specific stimulus or that we only use 10% of its capacity is simply not supported. (Beyerstein 1999).

MacLean's outdated model offered a hierarchy of function as layers of complexity were added as we move up the evolutionary tree. In essence, the cortex was doing the important, rational and creative thinking and potentially facing interruption from the limbic centre through the emotions that it can generate. This is a top-down model that fails to accommodate the brain's primary purpose. That number one priority is to survive both as an individual and as a species. Of course, we can theorise and predict (think?) and can capitalise on this extended function to achieve amazing things. However, even these abilities are subordinate to the overarching need to detect and mitigate actual or perceived threat.

This probably seems somewhat reductionist and perhaps rather utilitarian. However, it does provide a basis for recognising that, under threat, networks that engage with immediacy and agency are likely to become dominant. Stress will be kick-started as a primary physiological mechanism that the brain executes in order to enhance our survival.

The following story will give some insights into how it operates. I rang up my local health centre to make a routine appointment for a blood test. Before speaking to a receptionist, I had to listen to the following message with no option of skipping it:

> Thank you for ringing the ******* Practice. The NHS is experiencing current and rising strain with declining GP numbers, rising demand, struggles to recruit and retain staff; this is having a knock on effect for patients. In addition, GP practices have been at the forefront of the NHS response to the Covid 19 outbreak delivering vaccine appointments and delivering

patient care throughout. For this reason, we may not be able to offer you a routine appointment with a GP or other clinician in the time- scale that you have become accustomed to. Be rest assured that if you have an emergency on the day, we will speak to you. If you are calling about a Covid booster our primary care networks are operating behind schedule because of staffing constraints. Please be rest assured that you will receive an invitation, but our staff will not be able to provide more information at this time… (January 2022)

When we listen to a message like that we may be cognitively responding to the message and thinking about what we will say when we finally speak to the receptionist. However, those networks with a primary role in securing our immediate safety are scanning all those negatives and threats. You can just hear them all; shortage of GPs, problems with recruitment and retention, rising demand, no appointments and staffing constraints. At its best, this is counterproductive as a welcome message and at the worst it is hinting at NHS apocalypse.

Our perceptions can get worse! Our monitoring networks will pick up negative words and phrases out of context and it often rejects qualifying words. For example, the phrase 'a bit of a disaster' will almost certainly be stripped back to the panic trigger word 'disaster'. Because these mechanisms' role is to protect, they also have a role of stimulating an active response. Because of this we will underscore negative and threat words. A failure on our part to take action will stimulate us to collect increasingly negative information in order to try and get us to make a response. Consider working in a toxic team, the experience of many.

These monitoring networks will usually urge an aggressive response or encourage us to leave the scene. Our rational processes will often counter it with; 'It might pass', 'I need the job', 'If I left how would I pay the mortgage?' and 'People will think that I am a failure'. The suppression of action which is being initiated and sustained sets up a toxic stress response and can start a journey to a dark place inhabited by stress, anger, addictions and symptoms such as poor sleep (Maggio et al. (2013)).

It is essential to recognise that many of the inputs to these network systems are subliminal in that they do not always register on our conscious radar. I live on the south coast and for many years worked in London. My commute took me northwards up the M3 motorway. I was enjoying my work and even the commute was not too tedious. It became a habit to take a break at the Fleet Service Station, handy before the final run into London. Months passed by when I could not put my finger on the negative mood change that followed taking these breaks. A good mood ebbed away and was replaced with an anxious and rather dispirited one. Eventually, I cracked it. In order to get to the toilets, I passed the shop with newspapers set out for sale. Though I was not stopping to read them, I was taking in the headlines in a sort of osmotic process. If any product is misnamed it is the 'newspaper'. They frequently specialise in negative hyperbole, crisis, tragedy, disaster, emergency, panic, meltdown and many more. TV does a similar job and even if it is on in the background you will pick up these trigger words. One morning I counted the word 'crisis' being used on a TV news bulletin eight times in five minutes. We will be affected by such incessant messaging.

Back to the M3, I made the decision to look away from these destructive headlines and my mood did not return.

LE STRESS

One of my all-time favourite movies must be *Raiders of the Lost Ark* (1981). Bizarrely, the hero's name Indiana was borrowed from that of a dog belonging to series creator George Lucas. This Alaskan Malamute was also the inspiration for the character Chewbacca in *Star Wars*. So, back to *Raiders of the Lost Ark*. In the opening sequence, the intrepid Dr Jones enters an ancient Peruvian temple to obtain a priceless gold idol. As he takes the idol, antiquated defence mechanisms are triggered: automated arrows fly and finally a large boulder is released and looks likely to crush him. A gripping narrative, but this is also a powerful metaphor for how the brain reacts under threat, or even imagined threat, as an acute stress response is initiated and progressively builds.

The word 'stress' has entered common usage, it is also frequently misunderstood. The way that many people use this term is almost as a parenthetical summary of a bad situation. This could be about workload, skill deficit, a toxic work atmosphere or perhaps a struggle with an overbearing line manager. Its usage is often extended to include physical symptoms, which people feel are linked, such as headaches, palpitations, generalised chest pains and heartburn.

In 1946, even the prestigious Collège de France, the academicians responsible for maintaining the purity of the French language, struggled for several days with the problem of defining stress. Subsequently they decided that a new word would have to be created and *'le stress'* was appropriated. This was quickly followed by its adoption in other European languages by *el stress*, *il stress*, *lo stress* and *der stress*. There were derivatives in Russian, Japanese, Chinese and Arabic. Stress is one of the very few words you will see preserved in English in these and in other languages that do not use the Roman alphabet.

Its contemporary usage is generally traced back to Hans Selye (1956). He was born in Vienna and later moved to America and then to Canada. His earlier work, for which he was nominated for a Nobel Prize in 1949, was on endocrinology. Selye later researched the changes in the endocrine system that followed when an organism was exposed to a stimulus or stressor. In his original writings, there is no bias towards stress being inherently malignant; it just is. Confusion over the translation of his work resulted in a negative spin being attached to the word. He identified stress as an essential and normal response to many everyday stimuli. In many situations it is the mechanism that gets us 'off the sofa'. Faced with the confusion over the usage of the word, he eventually coined the terms 'eustress' for its positive operation and 'distress' for its negative twin.

Even this cursory exploration of the rapid changes in our neural processing suggests that, as human beings, our brains are seldom on idle. Perhaps all too often we push our brains beyond their safe operating limits. Because our brains can operate at such an amazing speed, it should not lead us to conclude that they should be utilised in such a relentless and over-demanding manner. Life is seldom straightforward, but if we lack an understanding of how our brains function as insistent organs of protection and survival and instead give undue status to our conscious thinking processes, our solutions and responses could range from the inappropriate to the downright disastrous.

This chapter concludes with the poem *'Beyond the Fear'* (Thomas, 2016). Its author, Will Thomas, is, like me, a coach and trainer who has undertaken a great deal of work in the educational sector and with individuals from many walks of life.

BEYOND THE FEAR...

Beyond the fear....
where your breath knows itself again
and the tightened straps of your panting ribs un-prison
your chest.

Your belly re-learns its past and your heart shifts
from panic-pump to
the valve-radio-receiver

of your soul.

The night-creep slows
and the spectres, bumps, and ghouls of the menacing
unknown
with their thousand twilight shocks re-configure
themselves...

As the cricket orchestra
toad-call,
shimmering-whisper of Silver Birch warmly forming in
the companion-forest

Where your mind makes friends
with the strangers of its own imagining finding new ways
of standing soft-knee'd

Where,
beyond the fear, freedom beckons.

(Reproduced by kind permission of the author).

2

IT'S DOING MY HEAD IN

Do not get me wrong, I would never trivialise mental health issues or the anguish that often walks alongside them. I did some work with the education department of a leading psychiatric hospital. There was always an awareness of the secured double doors that separated me from some of their deeply disturbed and disturbing adolescent patients. One story that will always remain with me was that of a teenage girl. Her mother had suffered bouts of serious depression and one day she took her young daughter to the top of the tower block where they were living. Grasping her daughter's hand, she jumped to her death. Right at the last moment, the girl managed to snatch her hand back and survived, at least physically. However, mentally she was severely traumatised and was sectioned and admitted as an inpatient in a secure unit. Her behaviour was extreme and it would be gratuitous to describe it. Individuals with such severe and harrowing psychiatric illness should always remain the remit of mental health professionals.

However, this book is about most people – those who experience depression or anxiety related symptoms. It is this group that much of the discussion on mental health is focused on in the media and in conversation. It is that group of us who often struggle with the pain of disconnection from relationships, become stripped of hope and develop the feeling that life might not reset.

Covid 19 was not the only pandemic. Following a systematic review, in an article published in *The Lancet* the writer concluded:

> We found that depressive and anxiety disorders increased during 2020 due to the COVID-19 pandemic. Even before the COVID-19 pandemic, depressive and anxiety disorders featured as leading causes of burden globally, despite the existence of intervention strategies that can reduce their effects. Meeting the added demand for mental health services due to COVID-19 will be difficult, but not impossible. Mitigation strategies should promote mental wellbeing and target determinants of poor mental health exacerbated by the pandemic, as well as interventions to treat those who develop a mental disorder. (Santamauro 2021, p.1701)

There are many would like to have first dibs in providing some resolution, whether from a compassionate stance or from the lucrative commercial possibilities of trying to resolve these widespread mental health issues. Mood changing medications have been prescribed on an industrial scale and talking therapies conscript ever more recruits into their practitioner ranks. For example, whilst the market dominating the Mental Health First Aid programme (MHFA) is provided by a community interest company, it is also extremely lucrative. In 2017, the organisation, commenting on its listing by the *Financial Times* in the 1,000 fastest-growing European companies, stated that:

> MHFA England provides courses teaching people to identify, understand and help a person who may be developing a mental health issue. The Community Interest Company's annual revenue has grown by 195% over the last three years, meaning the not-for-profit business is placed at number 547

on the list as compiled by data provider Statista. Entry into the list is only available for companies with revenue of at least €1.5m generated in 2015, which are headquartered in one of 31 European countries.

Nothing to date has proved to be the hoped-for magic bullet for our burgeoning mental health / wellbeing problems.

Antidepressants enjoy a partial success (this will be explored in more detail in a later chapter – *Breaking Bad*). The much-vaunted Cognitive Behaviour Therapy (CBT) has faltered. The latter was seen as a straightforward, quick and relatively inexpensive solution to many suffering with mental health issues. In a meta study that analysed 70 papers published between 1977 and 2014, researchers Johnsen and Friborg (2015) concluded that the effectiveness of CBT had reduced by roughly 50%. It is now half as effective in treating depression as it used to be. It may be that its rapid rise has resulted in too many inexperienced practitioners working in the field. Some have concluded that it could have worked as a placebo and that we now have a serious case of 'The Emperors Clothes'. Even Johnsen and Friborg have expressed concerns that publishing their paper might undermine CBT by damaging people's belief and trust in it as a treatment and, in turn, make matters worse by lowering expectations. The National Institute for Health and Care Excellence (NICE) are still advocates. On their website they offer the following statement as a summary for treating mild to moderate depression:

> Possible first treatments for mild to moderate depression include a self-help programme, a treatment called computerised cognitive behavioural therapy and a physical activity programme (exercise). These are described in the table on initial treatments

for mild to moderate depression. If you decide not to have these treatments or they are not available, you may be offered cognitive behavioural therapy (CBT for short) in a group with other people who have similar problems (see the table on psychological treatments for depression). (NICE 2009)

It is worth reflecting that if many medical and surgical units in our hospitals matched this level of performance that they would be investigated or even closed.

This is all shaping up as a bit of a Catch 22 situation; there is an increasing incidence of mainstream mental health issues such as stress and anxiety running parallel with a somewhat erratic range of solutions. Is there a way through? Perhaps the following observation by Rottenberg (2014) brings a useful focus:

> Expect no magic pill. One lesson learned from treating chronic pain is that it is tough to override responses that are hardwired into the body and the mind. Instead, we must follow the economy of mood where it leads, attending to the sources that brings so many into low mood states-think routines that feature too much work and too little sleep. We need broader mood literacy and an awareness of tools that interact with low mood states before they morph into longer more severe ones. These tools include altering how we think the events around us, our relationships, and conditions in our body. (Rottenberg, 2014, p. 32)

OVERVIEW

My own research into the provision of mental health and support in secondary schools (Coates and Bingham, 2020) showed that, in those that we studied there was certainly a response to concerns around the mental health of students and staff. However, there was little if any coherent thinking that structured the responses being offered. Anecdotal exploration of the responses available to support adults to achieve good mental health is not appearing to show a step change either.

The following model offers a way in to understand of the foundations of our mental health/wellbeing and how to secure good personal outcomes if we do start to mentally degrade. Perhaps. Even more importantly, we can use it to sidestep these issues from the get-go.

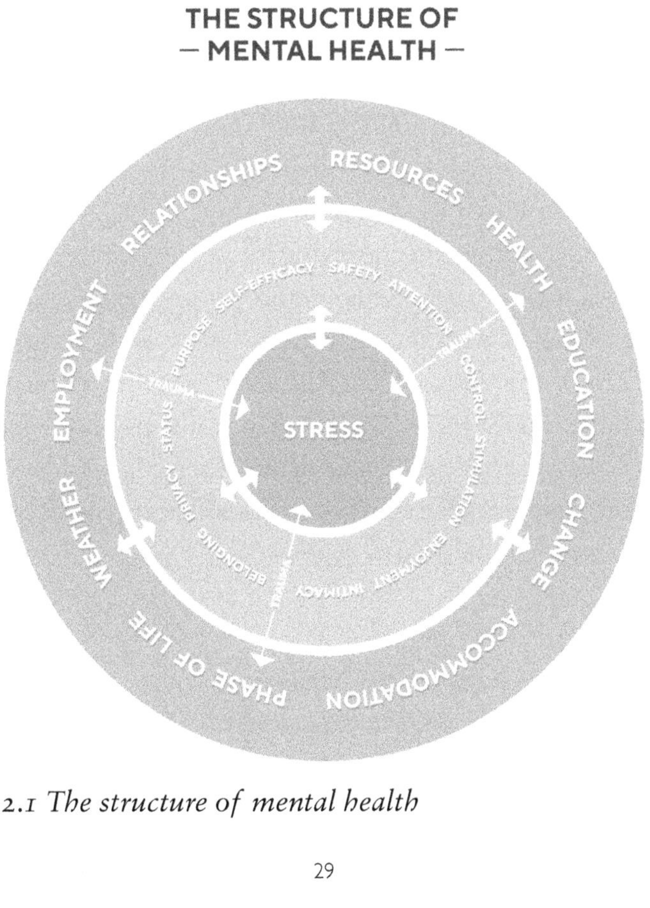

**THE STRUCTURE OF
— MENTAL HEALTH —**

Fig. 2.1 The structure of mental health

The best place to start unpacking this model is that middle band. This considers essential human needs. If we had no awareness of our needs and took no action to secure them then we would probably die of thirst or starve, fail to take shelter and not avoid dangerous situations. We would certainly not have skin in the survival game. This entry level awareness of our basic needs has been very much part of mankind's mental toolkit since the emergence of *homo sapiens*. In fact, many similar to ours are shared with other species.

Maslow, as far back as 1943, presented his well-known hierarchical model with physiological needs as being foundational and then topping it off with self-actualisation, his anthropocentric cherry on the top. An exploration of needs has driven a wide range of literature. It underpins much of the work by Seligman on Positive Psychology, probably CBT which is mentioned above, and popularist views on motivation such as Al Gore's one-time speech writer Pink (2009).

The model that we are unpacking is less hierarchical. Maslow perceived lower order needs require to be significantly met before engaging with the next level. This agenda of needs is drawn from the work of The Human Givens Institute and is more fluid. It is the work of psychologists and psychotherapists Griffin and Tyrrell (2003) They call their list *primal needs*. These foundational needs, the conclusion from their extensive clinical work can be summarised as follows:

- *Routinely feel safe*
- *Able to give and receive attention*
- *Have a sense of some control and in influence over events in life*
- *Feel stretched and stimulated by life to avoid boredom*
- *Feel life is enjoyable*

- *Experience intimacy with at least one other human being*
- *Have a feeling of belonging to a wider community*
- *Have the facility to have privacy and time for personal reflection*
- *Have a sense of status and a reasonably defined role in life*
- *Have a sense of self-efficacy (personal competence)*
- *Have a sense of meaning and purpose.*

There is no standardised value that can be given to each of these needs. It is not like measuring blood pressure or sugar levels where we can take a measurement and then check it against a table of normal. We each afford them something of a personal priority and a sense of what needs to happen for them to be met in our own lives. Their clinical practice is based on all human emotional difficulties stemming from chronically failing to meet one or more of these primal emotional needs (Tyrell 2015).

I suspect most of us could read the last sentence of the previous paragraph without breaking step. Surely, we all know what emotions are, for example: anger, fear, disgust, happiness and joy. If you start reading contemporary publications by psychologists on this subject, you will find that you have just fallen down a rabbit hole. There are a wide range of views on the subject and ironically the scientific protagonists of the various theories themselves get quite emotional on the subject. So, for now, park emotions and accept that when our fundamental or primal needs are not met there is a release of energy in the brain, a redirection of our thinking and our behaviours which may or may not resolve the problem. Conversely, when these primal needs are met a cocktail of neurotransmitters provide feelings of contentment and happiness. Our brains then have the capacity to turn to different things and change their perspective.

You can always tell a stressed person, but you probably cannot tell them much. Their thinking increasingly collapses into a world of sharp contrast with intermediate shades. Their speech is 'all or nothing' for example, 'It is always like this', 'Everyone ignores me', 'Nothing ever goes right for me'. When we are highly stressed potential options start to disappear.

At the core of this model is stress. This can operate appropriately, as when we go down a zip wire or if we are rock climbing; it can serve to energise us when we are problem solving or taking a penalty kick. It is usually an asset if we fall or are under immediate threat. It is less beneficial when it manifests as road rage or domestic violence. However, much of what will be considered is best understood in terms of the sustained and pernicious stress that drives our physiology and turns the tables on all our thinking and decision making. It is where the mechanism of stress is being triggered by complex and extended circumstances. This kind of immersive stress is illustrated by the case study of Daniel in the next chapter.

The outer circle of Fig. 2.1 details some aspects of our lived experience. You could probably add to the list. It is here that we usually turn to get our needs met but of course these same life events can also create a deficit on our primal needs. Quality relationships can meet our need for intimacy, contribute to our feelings of safety, provide an opportunity to give and receive attention, be enjoyable and even be part of our sense of meaning and purpose. Flipped they can be threatening, destabilise our sense of control, diminish that experience of intimacy and strip us of our sense of belonging. Life experiences that are so good can rapidly sour but then the converse is true – they can be changed to help us meet our needs and enhance our mental health.

The interplay can be complex. Our need for intimacy could express itself as being obsessive, or a desire for status can slip into becoming egotistical and our need for some level of control can morph into our becoming controlling.

Our brains lead a somewhat sheltered life; they exist in the darkened confine of the skull and construct meaning from the electrical and chemical inputs they receive. So often we misunderstand our experiences with and our reactions to people. We interpret our world through our own internal modelling and beliefs, frequently defending our stance or own brand of thinking.

This routine defence of our own position or beliefs is called 'Confirmation Bias'. It will be considered in greater detail in *Chapter 11 – Hall of Mirrors*. Several pieces of research found that despite being presented with a variety of evidence there was little change in the views of members of the two groups as they were presented with evidence. Participants in returning to their biased conclusions found ways to discard rational information in order to sustain their own position. Contradictory evidence was simply downplayed or discarded.. So perhaps Shakespeare nailed it after all:

> There is nothing either good or bad but thinking makes it so.
> William Shakespeare, *Hamlet*, Act 2 scene 2

THE WILD CARD

In the model there are arrows connecting our lived experience and the inner stress core. This is where the intensity of the experience is overwhelming and comes to take a pole position in our memories. This trauma, and it is not just the realm of people who have served in war zones or emergency services where it is often diagnosed as Post Traumatic Stress Disorder (PTSD), becomes memory that is insistent and persistent. The event does not get consigned to historical memory like holidays or changing jobs but serves to provide an intense and ever-present reference point as to what we have experienced and what is to us an extreme threat. It is deep rooted so that a soldier who has witnessed atrocities in Afghanistan cannot always dial down this threat marker when they have returned to the safety of the UK.

THE JOURNEY

There is a need to change our understanding of how our brain gathers and processes our context and get a handle on the fact that some of our lifestyle choices will impose a deficit on our primal needs. It is imperative that we come to terms with the nature of stress and its role in our mental health.

Sometimes the changes that we need to make are extensive and urgent. Often, the beneficial changes can be more marginal, but they do add up surprisingly quickly. Whatever they are, we owe it to ourselves to be more than a victim.

3

A PERFECT STORM

Meteorologists see perfect in strange things, and the meshing of three completely independent weather systems to form a hundred-year event is one of them. My God, thought Case, this is the perfect storm. (Junger, The Perfect Storm, 1997, p. 1)

The quotation comes from a book about the Halloween Nor'easter storm that led to the loss of a Nova Scotia fishing boat, the *Andrea Gail*. Case, the meteorologist quoted by Junger above, concluded that three different weather-related phenomena combined to create a perfect storm. Subsequently, the term has been used as a metaphor to refer to a disastrous situation caused by the intersection of multiple causes. It was widely used to describe the financial crisis of 2007-2012. It also works well as a title for the biographical disaster that forms the backbone of this chapter. The context is a school, but it could have been drawn from any number of situations. The story unfolds of a prevailing culture gorging itself on intended strategy and nearly destroying an individual in the process. Names have obviously been changed.

Daniel accepted the job as the headteacher of a medium-sized comprehensive school on the south coast. The area consisted of pockets of considerable affluence alongside much more modest, even deprived rural communities. Many of the surrounding villages demonstrated a fierce individualism, which would have inspired Steinbeck. The school had struggled for a number of years with the ability profile of its intake and had been top-sliced by competition from two nearby single-sex high schools still basking in the afterglow of earlier days as selective grammar schools. The loss of the school's sixth form, eight years previously, had conferred relegation status to the school in the eyes of both stakeholders and the community. This had been compounded by the school using marketing campaigns focused on the strapline of being a 'caring school'. An unfortunate side effect of this statement was that it was seen as being a synonym for providing for children with learning difficulties. The school became overloaded with such students, many of whom were steered towards it by the principals of the other more 'successful' local schools who did not want a potentially grade deflating intake.

The leadership of the school had been weak for a number of years. The previous principal had undertaken a range of worthy but unrelated civic duties at the expense of the effective running of the school. Much of the day-to-day running had been left in the hands of a willing vice-principal who was strong on bureaucracy, such as timetabling and rotas, but considerably less well-informed about the wider and rapidly evolving educational context. Daniel's predecessor had been pensioned off, leaving behind a legacy of unresolved problems.

The context and circumstances of the school had led to a culture where mediocrity was commonplace. Staff and even some of the advisors from the Local Education Authority (LEA) had come to understand the school as a victim. Advancing by a frame of even a few years this school would have been taken over by an academy chain.

The staff repeatedly challenged the burgeoning use of data. As one middle leader commented on being shown the data, 'What can you expect with these types of children?'. At a stroke, the clear diagnosis of underachievement was dismissed, and the professional emasculation of that staff member and his associates was confirmed. They were committed to coasting.

Daniel was convinced that this job was not a poisoned chalice and accepted the post and the challenge. He was encouraged to find a small but vocal minority of his colleagues who were both optimistic about the future and committed to bringing about constructive change.

On arrival, there were pressing issues. These included resolving costly overstaffing, some key problems around building maintenance and resourcing. A particularly pressing need was to deal with the school's deficit budget. The governors had sanctioned the latter on the basis of the belief that one of the deputy heads would be successful in finding another job and that pupil numbers would rise with income linked to the increase. Arguably, these were not inspired financial strategies and so one of Daniel's first tasks was to oversee making one of the two deputy headteachers redundant. This, in the end, proved to be the bureaucratic timetabler.

So, having secured today, Daniel started on tomorrow. He had read widely on the theory and research into school improvement. There was lots of good advice and case studies available and he had experience from a previous headship.

Implementing a process of change to affect both the raising of pupil achievement and changing culture requires considerable teamwork. However, few school leaders are afforded the luxury of building their own teams. Daniel was no exception, and had to work with the 'sitting tenants', most of whom had been appointed during the principal's interregnum to fill gaps in the capacity of the leadership of the school. The governors were strong advocates for these people continuing in their roles. He soon realised that this leadership team were short on both capability and capacity. However, with a limited budget there was little room to make changes. There were obviously professional development issues, which had to be addressed. This was seen as part of his role and was factored into his overall strategic planning, which was appropriately configured over a five-year period. Key to the success of this strategic plan was to secure the engagement and commitment of this team to become active advocates and executors of the plan.

It was at this point that the factors that were to shape the perfect storm began to emerge. Much of what was to take place had its roots in the very members of this leadership team, the school governors and their separate and joint duplicity. The school had a full complement of governors with a grasp of politics but with a lamentable lack of understanding of education. A faultline running through the middle of the governing body further intensified their dysfunction. One half was made up of a group of rich and extremely rich retired business executives. The other half were from a less advantaged socio-economic group, many of whom were elected as parent governors. The control lay with the affluent whilst the frustration was with the other group. There was a continuous conspiracy by the elite core to disenfranchise the others by withholding information or by browbeating them into submission in meetings. The governance of the school was not a support but a disabling and suppurating sore.

So, returning to the team, a pen portrait of each of its members would be essential in understanding what was about to unfold:

Daniel (Headteacher). Newly appointed to the role but having completed a successful headship of another school. He was well qualified at a postgraduate level in school leadership and had the practical understanding of both running a school and the process of raising achievement.

Fiona (Deputy Headteacher). Stylish and politically astute, though very much more at the Machiavellian rather than the Mandela end of the political spectrum. The persona that was routinely projected was maternal; she was everybody's agony aunt. Upon Daniel's appointment she made overtures of support together with a pledge of personal commitment to the task of turning the school round. Two points were to emerge. First, she only undertook those tasks that appealed or which gave her public recognition. She would sidestep confrontational situations, for example, always finding excuses to avoid lesson observations with the challenge of feedback to the teacher. Behind the pleasant image was an accomplished plotter and schemer with a social network penetrating the governors and the wider educational authority. During a long period when Fiona was absent following a fall at home, Daniel was surprised to receive a text from a valued middle leader saying 'Be careful: Fiona considers this to be her school. Even though she is absent, she is engineering your downfall'. On speaking to the colleague, they said they would not say more and did not wish to be involved. Further investigation revealed that Fiona had actively manipulated the previous headteacher's resignation and stage managed her early retirement. This she had accomplished by inviting the senior secondary advisor from the LEA for supper, and over the meal she had undertaken an adroit professional assassination of this headteacher. Daniel was to discover this, three years into post, and find that old habits die hard.

Paul (Assistant Headteacher). Paul's key responsibility was raising standards at Key Stage 4. There was certainly a capability issue with little contemporary knowledge of this area and again a marked avoidance of working directly with staff. There was also a darker side. When Daniel had just taken up his post, in fact at the end of the first week, he had had to hold a disciplinary meeting relating to Paul having obstructed a 14-year-old girl from leaving his office. This had led to a parental complaint. Daniel, generous (perhaps over generous) by nature, had decided this was an aberration. Subsequently, he discovered that Paul had made advances to several female staff. One had left because of his inappropriate harassment, which included leaving notes on her windscreen. Sadly, Daniel only found out later and, even then, only accidently. Exploring the situation further it became apparent that he was almost universally disliked by staff and perceived as being lazy and self-serving.

John (Assistant Headteacher). A former head of maths in the school, he had moved into senior leadership on the 'data ticket'. Undoubtedly competent in this area, which was also happened to be one that Daniel felt less secure with, it gave him an edge over his headteacher. Creative by style and one of the few forward-thinking members of staff, he brought a valued intellectual dimension to the school's leadership team. Some considerable time later his lack of personal integrity surfaced. His style with staff was coercive to the point of being intimidating. His bullying attitude was the basis of a number of complaints by female staff to the point where it precipitated an outstanding female head of maths to resign her post. Much later Daniel was told in confidence that John was opening his emails in advance.

Gillian (Head of English). A consummate professional who was much respected by other colleagues. Under the pressure of being put down by other members of the team and confused by the duplicity she witnessed, she no longer felt able to contribute to leadership meetings.

Andy (Community Lead). A pleasant individual who was verbally supportive though with a tendency not to walk the talk. Many staff perceived him as work shy and consequently he was not widely respected. There were repeated rumours that he was having an affair with the wife of the vice-chair of governors. Whilst this was never substantiated, it inevitably had an impact upon the disdain with which he was viewed.

Daniel tried to concentrate on taking the school forward and rebuilding its tarnished reputation, though he repeatedly deviated from his intentions in the face of other pressures. A great deal of time was spent campaigning for resources, recruiting staff, responding to an unsupportive governing body and dealing with too many pastoral issues left unresolved by Fiona. Many of the teaching staff were not classroom effective and required intensive management to drag them out of an earlier educational dispensation. He became overstretched and lacked adequate support from any quarter. Even the LEA senior advisor could only come up with the suggestion of a core transformational strategy for the school that we should change the uniform to striped blazers from plain blue!

Returning to the central metaphor, a challenging situation was now moving towards the perfect storm. The first weather front rolling in: Fiona, the deputy headteacher was off work for a significant period following an accident. The budget did not allow for a replacement and there was also a lack of capacity within the school to provide effective cover. The absence was of unpredictable length, making contingency plans problematic. In the end, she was absent for a year. John, the assistant headteacher, saw the problems as an opportunity for personal advancement. His apparent help ran in parallel with a plan to undermine Daniel. He assumed a dominant, often bullying approach to staff at all levels. Matters were exacerbated when he suffered a neurological event before the December of Daniel's last year. After a short absence, he became increasingly malignant, though charming to Daniel's face. This was the time when his behaviour precipitated the resignation of the head of maths. John adopted a high-risk strategy, which ultimately had a devastating impact on the leadership of the school. Responsible for the school's timetable, he met with Daniel weekly to explore this against the demands of the curriculum, budget and staffing. This had been routine practice for some four years. These meetings, together with reports of consultations with middle leaders, sounded completely plausible. In late May, he published the teaching timetable for the following year and it became clear that he had used an IT program which, whilst providing a starting point for generating a timetable, produced something completely unworkable in practice. The chair of governors was apoplectic and wanted him sacked there and then. Unexpectedly, a week later the focus of criticism changed to Daniel with John inexplicably being excused. It emerged that there was an intrinsic linkage between the two through a shared membership of an exclusive club. This completely turned the tables.

In all probability, Daniel should have monitored the development of the timetable more closely, but his teaching load had increased to nearly 50%. This because of the need to dismiss a member of staff following a pupil assault. He was the only staff member with that curriculum speciality and efforts to appoint an appropriate supply teacher had been unproductive. Teaching this much is unheard of for a secondary headteacher, in fact, many do not teach at all.

A further challenge coincided with this as the site manager suffered a heart attack and was ultimately invalided out of the post. Again, temporary solutions proved limited because of financial constraints and Daniel ended up locking up the secondary school and setting the alarm for three nights a week, often after evening lettings. This carried on for nearly six months.

The return of the deputy headteacher from nearly a year of absence brought neither support nor respite for Daniel but rather further demonstrations of her destructive political manoeuvring.

The strands had coalesced, and the perfect storm was now a reality. Support from any source was entirely absent. He had aired these problems with the chair of governors and LEA staff who showed a committed disinterest. Discussions with those who should have provided support deteriorated into an increasingly surrealist dialogue.

It is important to understand that Daniel, in common with all of us, did not have compartmentalised brains – all of life is there. Alongside the toxic work-related issues, he also had a young family, financial demands, a challenging commute, household maintenance, ageing parents, health concerns and family bereavement. Not all aspects of life were problematic, but they were all clamouring for headspace.

One morning Daniel went into the school and sat at his desk. He looked down to see large droplets of water on his desk blotter and realised these were not from a roof leak but his tears. This was the overture to a sustained period of depressive illness even to the point of contemplating suicide. It began to cycle as an increasing range of foundational needs. After all, he now self-branded himself as a failure. His family stretched salary was coming to an end with the potential repossession of his house very much in view. He did not return to working as a headteacher. With appropriate help, he did manage to pull back from the abyss, though it was a further five years before he enjoyed personal stability.

The school? The local authority eventually realised their neglect and incompetency and poured resources into the school. Ironically these enabled the implementation of the strategic plan that Daniel had crafted.

I have worked as a coach for twenty years and could give parallel examples relating to individuals working as; solicitors, company directors, clergy, healthcare professionals, teaching assistants, property developers, trainers, pilots, academics and people running small businesses. The list is a long as the people that I have encountered. Most roles are complex and often ill-defined. There is a sense of the football manager about them; a run of 'lost games' and suddenly the individual's employment is terminated. Our work is set in the context of rapid changes: technology, globalisation and international instability. Personal relationships are more ephemeral and breakdown in them is commonplace. People embrace complexity in their lives or have that complexity imposed and reach a point where their resources become overstretched. Many will be aware of the metaphor of the frog in the slowly heating water which does not recognise the rise in temperature and slowly boils to death unaware of its circumstances. This is a great metaphor even though it is overused. It certainly describes the predicament many find themselves in. It is such a shame that it has been exposed as an urban myth, though sadly the experience and consequences of prolonged and excessive stress on individuals are far from being a fable.

4

DID I MENTION STRESS?

In 2003 I went on a sponsored bike ride around Northern Tanzania. Cycling through the bush along a rough track, I suddenly realised that I was not alone and that this was not part of the Longleat Safari Park. Two ostriches were converging on the same path. This was the equivalent of over 2000 chicken nuggets travelling towards me at around 40mph. It was concerning, to say the least, but fortunately at the last moment they veered away. However, what was fascinating was the way that my physiology moved so rapidly onto 'turbo boost'. My body was flooded with adrenaline from glands on the top of my kidneys. The blood drained from my body surface to service my major muscle groups. Less obvious was the cortisol, again from my adrenal glands. This steroid was bathing my joints to give protection against potential damage. I was ready for action. With hindsight, there was a dawning realisation that cycling around the UK had not entirely equipped me for this potentially terminal moment.

My physiological response to this threat is pretty standard stuff which most people know: classic flight or fight. We are also aware of that shaky climbdown as the immediate threat recedes, usually after about 27 minutes. This rapid survival response is initiated by the paired amygdala, perhaps, our brain's smoke detectors. They, however, do more than emit an irritating high-pitched noise. There is a chain of events that travels rapidly from the base of the brain (hypothalamus) and things move quickly onwards through to the adjacent pituitary gland and on to the adrenal glands which are on the top of the kidneys. It is these glands that secrete the adrenaline and cortisol. They set us up for action but also have a significant effect on our thinking bringing about a blinkered focus. This is often referred to as the Hypothalamus/Pituitary Gland/Adrenal Gland Axis (HPA Axis). As they circulate, we are less likely to consider options and increasingly focus on survival.

Perhaps less clear to many people is that this same mechanism can be activated and importantly sustained, by circumstances less immediately dramatic than cycling with poultry. The argument has been made that we have a set of primal needs and if these are not met the brain will focus on actions to resolve this. We will barely notice feeling a bit thirsty, a need easily met with a cup of tea. However, the onset of serious dehydration will up the game considerably. Similarly, feeling a bit put upon at work might be seen as an irritation, whereas being continuously criticised by an overbearing line manager or being bullied or believing that we are not valued is going to impact our need for status, meaning and a sense of belonging, security or community. The former is likely to pass with the lunchbreak or the weekend, the latter will persist and probably build as our brain gathers more and more negative supporting evidence as it attempts to get us to take action. The brain is detecting threat and triggering the HPA but the endocrine response will not be going away anytime soon.

There is no doubt that this chronic rather than acute operation of the endocrine system, with its production of adrenaline and cortisol, is detrimental to health. It can serve as a significant precursor to serious health issues. Tyrrell (2007) suggests that sustained stress is a greater predictor of coronary heart disease than moderate drinking, moderate obesity and even moderate smoking. Though, of course, no recommendation is being made that these three should be adopted as an alternative to stress.

I would argue that such a sustained stress-driven physiological state is likely to have a significant and detrimental impact upon both our physical and our mental health. If indeed, these two can be divided. The Cortisol will start to degrade our memories even chipping away at one of the key areas associated with memory, the hippocampus. Our thinking will narrow, reducing creative possibilities as we tend to generate defensive/aggressive responses towards our situation and others involved in it. This will be explored in more detail in later chapters; it is, however, self-evident, that such changes in our thought processes are unlikely to be beneficial. The psychologist Csikszentmihalyi (1990) argues along similar lines with his identification of a preferential optimal state, which he terms 'flow'. This is calm creative thinking as opposed to monochrome survival thinking. It is fascinating to listen to highly stressed people using all or nothing phrases; *'It always happens to me'*, *'What else can I expect'* and *'There is no way out of this'*. Hormone-driven, our minds will cycle as we try to find our way out of our problem maze. Depression will be a frequent consequence of such intense rumination. Beneficial sleep patterns will be an early victim to this fractured mindset.

This was Daniel's circumstance in the previous chapter as the situation became increasingly difficult to resolve. Day by day his primal needs were moving into deficit:

- *Status*: This is diminishing as his tenure of the post was being questioned.
- *Purpose*: He was a committed professional. He understood his job as a vocation and now his values-driven occupation began to crumble.
- *Self-efficacy*: We need to have some experience of competency in our roles. This was now fading as his hard-earned skills were failing to resolve the situation.
- *Control*: Events began to spiral out of his grasp as key people started to plot his downfall.
- *Enjoyment*: Working to provide a quality education for young people had always given him a great deal of enjoyment. This was becoming increasingly soured by events.
- *Safety*: As his employment came under threat, his health began to deteriorate, and he became increasingly concerned about supporting his family. Meetings at work began to feel like bear baiting with him in the title role.
- *Belonging:* He began to feel increasingly pushed to the periphery of the organisation. His challenging situation was degenerating into a place of bleak isolation.
- *Intimacy*: The situation was no longer left at the school entrance. Worry and anxiety was invading his family life and relationships and these were becoming strained.
- *Privacy:* An opportunity for peace and reflection can be refreshing. However, faced with such a toxic situation, being alone now intensified his perceptions of threat. You are never alone with a problem.

The situation has rapidly become a black run of stress and definitely not in a good way.

FROZEN

Many people know about the flight and fight adrenaline driven stress response. There is another option that can be triggered by threat. This has been highlighted by Porges (2017) and developed as his Polyvagal Theory. This is more rooted in research than that term might suggest. It is centred around the function of the vagus nerve. This has a key role in regulating functions such as our digestion, heart rate, and breathing. It cuts in with reflex actions such as coughing, sneezing, swallowing, and vomiting. Additionally, it has a role in controlling the muscles behind facial expressions. What we are feeling is, after all, usually displayed on our faces and in the sound of our voices. Without the vagus nerve it is unlikely that we would be able to tell how anyone else was feeling.

A bit of anatomy. Nerves are usually insulated with myelin, a largely fatty substance that ensures that the electrical messages travel from source to destination without detour. This insulation also helps speed up transmission rates. Porges (2017) concluded that rather than just being a simple linear nerve, the vagus nerve is more of a system and has three components. The oldest of these in is the dorsal vagal, a bit of an evolutionary leftover, which has no myelin sheath. If this operates when a situation of threat feels uncontrollable and we are feeling overwhelmed then it will initiate a freeze or shut down. This parallels the way that reptiles can become immobile when stressed. A second more structurally complex nerve, complete with an insulating myelin sheath, can come into play initiating our fight and flight response. These nerves are part of the sympathetic nervous system prompting action, though the operating priority of the two is not always apparent. There is a third part of the system, the ventral vagal, which is the more highly evolved and complex and is part of our parasympathetic nerve system, which comes into its own when threat recedes. This myelinated nerve supports our social communication and engagement system and moderates our heart rate and breathing. It is also involved in our hearing, the operation of our facial muscles and speech and tonality. It settles us down and actually conserves our energy resources.

For some this a bit out there. Some, such as Grossman and Taylor (2007), have suggested that Porges work does not hold up. In turn, Porges (2021) offers a robust rebuttal of their challenge. Nearly 30 years on, Polyvagal theory continues to gain traction in areas such as autism, trauma and work in the field of counselling. My own interest came from working with a group, headed by rheumatologist Dr. Chris Moran, trying to find some resolution to the largely implacable problems of Chronic Fatigue Syndrome / Fibromyalgia and found that this theory provided some glimmers of hope.

The following quotation from Porges (2011) provides a useful perspective on our nervous system's actions to moderate our potentially overriding defensive mechanisms:

> "Playing nice" comes naturally when our neuroception detects safety and promotes physiological states that support social behaviour. However, pro-social behaviour will not occur when our neuroception misreads the environmental cues and triggers physiological states that support defensive strategies. After all, "playing nice" is not appropriate or adaptive behaviour in dangerous or life-threatening situations. In these situations, humans – like other mammals – react with more primitive neurobiological defence systems. To create

relationships, humans must subdue these defensive reactions to engage, attach, and form lasting social bonds. Humans have adaptive neurobehavioral systems for both pro-social and defensive behaviours." (p12)

MIND GAMES

In Spielberg's *The Bridge of Spies* (2015) the principal characters; Donovan (Tom Hanks) and Abel (Mark Rylance) have a repeated dialogue.

> Donovan asks, 'Aren't you worried?'
> Abel makes the reply 'Would that help?'

Donovan is intrigued by Abel's resignation to events. Perhaps that curiosity is fuelled by it not being a common response. Would quoting that screenplay to someone who is on the edge help? Probably not, and the individual's issues and associated charged state are not likely to be stopping anytime soon. Worry, anxiety and their kissing cousin depression are likely to include rumination in the mix. Challenging situations can feel relentless and without much likelihood of obtaining a good outcome. The stress response generated from such a demanding circumstance is not easily dialled down and is likely to be pressed into extended service, something for which it was never intended.

We have evolved with a further powerful survival tool, the ability to anticipate and predict events. If we can anticipate a threat in advance of having to confront it, then that makes huge sense. When driving it is better to anticipate the possibility of a child running into the road because we are near a school and it is around 8.45am rather than performing an emergency stop as a child steps out between parked vehicles. Top seeded tennis players receiving a serve in excess of 140mph cannot continuously track the ball from opponent to their own response. They are great athletes but are also exceptional in their ability to predict how tennis balls travel. When you are thirsty and drink a large glass of water, your feelings of thirst diminish. Strangely, this satiation of our thirst anticipates the actual physiological changes which will not happen for a further 20 minutes.

We also apply this predictive ability to complex situations such as those found at work or in relationships. This can work against us, and when we experience sustained stress the more likely it is that our ability to predict can malfunction and even become unstable. This is particularly the case in the focus that we give to aspects of our story and also in terms of the way that we assemble our individual subplots as we generate our narrative. When we are stressed our internal as well as our external narratives can move from positive to negative extremely quickly.

STRESSED TO KILL

Self–help books are big business, Walker (2019) writing for the Guardian newspaper commented:

> Sales of self-help books have reached record levels in the past year, as stressed-out Britons turn to celebrities, psychologists and internet gurus for advice on how to cope with uncertain times.
>
> Three million such books were sold – a rise of 20% – according to figures from Nielsen Book Research, propelling self-improvement or pop psychology into one of the fastest-growing genres of publishing.

That is even before the Covid Pandemic.

Experience is universal and information is cheap but taking ideas beyond anecdote and opinion is altogether more demanding. In exploring what is currently being published on stress, I came across a book presenting it as being significantly positive McGonical (2015). I have never argued that stress is wholly detrimental but rather that sustained stress, linked to a threatening context and powered by a negatively leaning personal narrative was a toxic mix.

Not surprisingly, I have paused and reflected on McGonical's optimistic perspective on stress. This is a Stanford based health psychologist who has huge book sales and over 12 million views of her TED Talk; *How to make stress your friend* (2013).

Of course, we do live in a world where there is an extensive menu of stressors; climate change, energy prices, delayed access to health care, extensive reformatting of our working practices, relationship breakdowns, the intrusion of social media and many more. Sustained stress is an important issue as wide-ranging health issues have been linked to it. For example, Tawakol et al. (2017) looked at and confirmed the established linkage between stress and heart disease. Could McGonical's conclusions be a solution to this or could they be inherently dangerous if we were now to ignore that cocktail of stress that many of us are routinely immersed in? The book relies on what is often described as positive psychology, though repackaged in her writing as 'mindset interventions'. Is she correct and should we now just accept that with some reframing of the narrative behind the stress all will be well or improved? Of course, reframing or interpreting events differently is a powerful and extremely useful tool but I would argue that its benefits are exaggerated in her advocacy. Surprisingly, she does not reference the seminal researchers in this area, the positive psychologists such as Seligman and Csikszentmihalyi (2000).

There is also an implied subliminal consequence of reading her book. McGonical states:

> When you put this book away, you likely won't have a clear sense yet of how its ideas will take root in your life. That's part of the magic of mindset interventions. If the science holds true, you might not even remember what this book is about (2015 p.222)

The hormones cortisol and adrenaline are, not surprisingly, frontrunners in her discussions about stress. Unexpectedly, McGonical elevates another hormone, oxytocin, to a prominent position. This hormone is more usually associated with childbirth and bonding. In the vernacular, it is sometimes referred to as the 'cuddle hormone' with a linkage to social connection. It certainly does have some role in stress reduction. In her arguments, it has somewhat photobombed the bigger picture associated with the two much more influential stress contributors.

McGonical states that she had identified with the majority of psychologists who believe that sustained stress is not just potentially, but actually harmful. The turning point for her appears to be when she came across a study by Keller et al. (2012). This is the same study referenced by Epstein (2015) as Witt in his withering critique. This study appears to suggest that if you believe that stress is harmful then it will have a detrimental impact on health and, where the individual embraces stress positively, it is not as harmful and that it can actually be harnessed as an asset.

The Keller et al. (2012) study was conducted over a number of years (longitudinal). Now, there is a foundational rule linked with research not to confuse 'correlation' and 'causality'. Consider the discovery that increasing numbers of butchers' shops is matched by finding an increased number of vegans in the same community. This is obviously absurd as neither of these causes an increase in the other. Self – evidently, they are both related to the population in a given community. Epstein offers a similar criticism of the way that McGonical has used this study:

> McGonigal credits a 2012 study by Whitney P. Witt, then at the University of Wisconsin–Madison, and her colleagues for her epiphany, but that study showed only that believing one's stressful experiences are harmful was correlated with illness and early mortality. That does not mean beliefs caused illness. There is a simpler, less mysterious way of accounting for the results; people who experience stress but who suffer minimal ill effects from it come to believe that stress cannot hurt them, whereas people who do suffer ill effects come to believe that stress is harmful. Voilà, we now have the correlation those researchers found but with belief as an outcome rather than a cause. McGonigal continues to make this type of error throughout her book. (2015, p. 70)

There are many writers and pundits out there who proffer solutions to the problems that we experience in our lives. It is important to make a careful assessment of what is being suggested and I include this book in that caveat as well. Perhaps with McGonigal, the clue lies less with her doctorate and its focus on humanistic medicine or her first degree in psychology but more with a further degree in mass communication. Her main role at Stanford is listed as teaching a course on Presentation and Communication Skills for Academics (Stanford 2021).

Despite this unexpected detour, I am going to stick with a more conventional view of stress. Again, this is by Barrett (2020):

> It's important to understand the human brain doesn't seem to distinguish between the different sources of chronic stress. If your body budget is already depleted by the circumstances of life like physical illness, financial hardship, hormone surges, or simply not sleeping or exercising enough, your brain becomes more vulnerable to stress of all kinds. This includes the biological effects of words designed to threaten, bully, or torment you or people you care about. When your body budget is continually burdened, momentary stressors pileup, even the kind that you normally bounce back from quickly. It's like children bouncing on the bed. The bed might withstand 10 kids bouncing at the same time, but the 11th one snaps the bedframe.
>
> Simply put, a long period of chronic stress can harm the human brain. Scientific studies are absolutely clear on this point. (p.91)

5

TOO MUCH, TOO FAR, TOO SOON OR TOO LONG

(The opening section contains descriptions of violence. You may wish to skip to the main body of the text).

There is an old and perhaps not particularly funny joke that a drummer is someone who hangs around with musicians. Not the case for a friend, Matt King, who is the Principal Percussionist with the Bournemouth Symphony Orchestra and also Professor of Percussion with the Royal Marines School of Music. If you listened to the Mission Impossible theme you will have sampled his work. However, he had the worst first day at work of anyone that I have ever met.

Matt enrolled as a cadet bandsman with the Royal Marines. Determined not to be late, he was in the barracks in Deal in plenty of time. At 8.22am on the 22nd September 1989, the Provisional Irish Republican Army exploded a time bomb at the Royal Marines' School of Music. The building collapsed. It destroyed the recreational centre and levelled an adjacent three-story building. Civilian homes nearby were damaged, and the blast was heard and felt in nearby Deal.

Some of the casualties were buried under the rubble for a number of hours. Heavy duty military lifting equipment had to be brought in to free them. Kent Ambulance Service had been on strike at the time of the blast but immediately volunteered to end their strike action in order to help. Eleven bandsmen were killed and twenty-two were injured. One body was eventually recovered from the roof of a nearby house.

Fortunately, most of the bandsmen who normally used the building as a barracks were already up and practising marching on the nearby parade ground when the blast occurred. These marines did witness the buildings collapsing and the death of their comrades.

Amongst those who witnessed the blast was recruit Matt King. In an instant, he had to respond to an existential threat accompanied by the visual images of carnage with the soundtrack of the bomb blast, the smell of the explosive and the grit of the dust cloud. In a state of profound shock, he had to involve himself in responding to the disasters. Many of the bandsmen who were not directly involved would also have been affected by survivor syndrome, that guilt that wrongly affects those whom a tragedy leaves behind. Head and Williams (2006) recorded the presence of these teenage recruits and the fact that they were in a state of shock for several days after. Good luck with that; trauma is seldom easily or quickly erased.

Military action is a rich source of such trauma. In World War ll the term lack of moral fibre (LMF) was used to describe RAF aircrew who were struggling to cope with their repeated combat missions. Individuals had to cope with the sheer fear, fatigue and horror of aerial warfare which was generating increasing numbers of psychological as well as physical casualties. In 1940 it was recommended that squadron commanders should identify those individuals who had lost their confidence as 'lacking in moral fibre'. This was an attempt to put clear blue water between them and those who had suffered the more acceptable physical injuries (Wells 2014). Subsequently, these men had their files stamped with a large red 'W'. This stood for 'waverer'. This was initiated to prevent the systemic problem of such psychological stress leaking out into the public domain! English (2008) records that 2,726 cases (including 2,337 Non-Commissioned Officers) were classified in this way.

This was punitive. Such a classification would strip a man of his flying badge and longer term from getting a well-paid job in civil aviation at the end of the war. Officers designated this way would lose their commissions and even the option of taking an alternative role as ground crew. The non-commissioned officers would be reduced to aircraftmen (2nd class) and given menial roles such as cleaning the latrines. At the end of the war these men could be drafted to work in the coal mines or conscripted to serve in the army.

Even accepting that these were exceptional times, these aircrew were exposed to horrendous levels of stress. Speaking of the experience of being a rear gunner in a Lancaster Bomber (Swan 2009) records:

> Having been in Cartwright's turret. That rear turret is the least enviable position in the Lanc. An attack almost inevitably comes from behind and the rear gunner receives the full cannon blast. Sometimes he's the only one who gets it, the Lanc. having started corkscrewing immediately on the attack and thereby escaping but in so many cases, too late to save the Gunner. Cartwright makes light of it saying that if he has to be housed out of the turret on return to base – as has happened on some occasions – at least he'll know nothing about it. (p. 28)

Witnessing such scenes and living with the anticipation of similar possibilities happening to themselves must inflict severe psychological damage. Fortunately, the term 'lacks moral fibre' has largely been consigned to history, to be replaced by the less judgemental, post-traumatic stress disorder (PTSD).

Aside from military action, many of us do experience life events which leave an indelible mark on the title page of our memories. Some are extreme such as domestic abuse, rape, a serious car accident, robbery or perhaps job loss. Recently, my wife and I went on a cruise around the Western Mediterranean. You can dine in aloof isolation. However, we enjoyed sharing a table with strangers. On day three at breakfast, one seasoned 'cruiser' immediately explained that he was a Liverpool fan. Actually, I had already spotted that from the overstretched letters on his football shirt. Almost without drawing breath, he explained that he was at the tragic Hillsborough game where Liverpool played Nottingham Forest and a crowd surge cost the lives of 97 fans. My fellow diner had found the dead body of a fellow fan across his feet. The urgency with which he needed to tell me this was a powerful indication of how imminent this memory was.

There is no sliding scale of impact; so something that might seem trivial to one person could be internalised as profound and disturbing by someone else. I was coaching a lady in her fifties and she shared that as a girl her parents had run a guest house, the kind that some people live in for extended periods. A few of the residents were down the more disreputable end of the spectrum of the population. When she was about seven, one lodger used to come in late and climb in through her bedroom window. They moved through her room to gain access to the main body of the house. She was adamant that nothing had happened to her. Her room was just a keyless entry point to their own rooms. However, this nocturnal visitor had left her with a lifetime legacy of anxiety.

So far, I have mainly considered trauma in individuals from directly experienced events. There are also risks when we are exposed to the second-hand accounts. Reflect on the impact on a social worker hearing about the extremes of abuse suffered by a small child from people who should have been compassionate parents or carers. McCann and Pearlman (1990) described this as vicarious trauma. The symptoms of vicarious trauma seem to be the same as those who have experienced real-time traumatic incidents.

My son and daughter-in-law have a great track record in buying me birthday presents. Standouts to date include an evening at the London O2 with Mark Knopfler and a pair of Croc shoes. This year has absolutely moved up a notch with an evening at the local theatre on the *Psychology of Serial Killers*. I am not sure what this says about their understanding of me. I will also be fascinated to see the rest of the audience. There may be one or two that encourage me to walk home along well-lit streets. In the publicity flyer it is described as 'Better than Netflix' and one person commented 'Incredible. I'll never sleep again'. So, I could be haunted and even disturbed by the presentation. It is possible that a second hand or even the invented narrative can take up residence in our amygdala.

The pathway to vicarious trauma for individuals such as counsellors, therapists, health care professionals, emergency service support personnel, teachers and social workers appears to be when they connect empathetically with their clients. This tends to happen where the latter are sharing personal and harrowing experiences with those tasked with professional listening (Naylor 2022) The focus of discussion around vicarious trauma has been mainly on the impact of such engagement by these skilled helpers. Research and discussion is continuing to evolve and writers in the field are recognising increasing parallels with the experiences found in the wider and less obviously traumatically exposed population. Following the 9/11 attack on the World Trade Center in the United States, many Muslims were stereotyped as terrorists and they suffered violent attacks. The feelings of insecurity and the potential threats experienced by many American Muslims caused individuals to suffer from vicarious trauma (Ashraf and Nassar 2018). That same study found that those with a strong sense of religious identity were even more likely to experience such vicarious trauma.

At the time of writing, the tragic war in Ukraine is continuing. Many people are being exposed to a daily diet of rolling news showing the impact of a brutal war. These images are often accompanied by distressing interviews with particularly vulnerable Ukrainian citizens who are suffering as a result of displacement, bereavement, injury or privation. There will be consequences from the sustained impact of such media immersion. It seems to have hit home to a greater extent than the no less horrific but more distant conflicts such as Syria or Afghanistan. Some people speak about becoming desensitised whilst others are haunted by the scenes of destruction delivered to our homes like some malignant takeaway.

When trauma invades our being, fixed penalty fines should be imposed on those found saying 'I know just how you feel', 'Snap out of it', 'Time is a great healer' and historic gems like 'Worse things happen at sea'. Such cliches are unlikely to excise trauma or even to turn down its insistent volume.

MEMORIES

So how did the young bandsman Matt King, along with so many others faced with such insistent experiences, begin to process what was happening? How do people deal with the often multi-sensorate experience of traumatic events? What happens when we are assaulted by circumstances that are too much, too far, too soon or too long?

Because the focus has often been on PTSD, discussions, in turn, have frequently been linked with the extremes witnessed and experienced by the armed forces and the emergency services. Perhaps because of this many of us feel uncomfortable claiming this ground for our own experiences that we believe to be more mundane. There has also been a range of terminology thrown into this complex mix: trauma, compassion fatigue (Adams, Boscarino and Figley 2006), PTSD and vicarious trauma. I would suggest that it is helpful to turn this semantic volume down. I propose talking in more general and perhaps more inclusive terms of trauma and argue for the following unifying theory. Doing this will help focus on applying common strategies for all types of trauma.

For a moment or two, think back over the last ten years and, hopefully, you have managed to have a few holidays in that time. See if you can remember some of them; where you went, who you went with, what the weather was like and perhaps how long you went for. My wife and I did this the other day and we got quite a lot of the details of our various holidays correct. We were a bit hazy whether went to Mallorca the year before we went to Portugal or the year after. With varying degrees of success and a few detours most of us will find that we have date-stamped these kinds of memories.

In a previous chapter, I suggested a flexible model of the brain based on interlinked networks. Even so, some areas still seem to have a more specialised role than others. Towards the back of the brain is the hippocampus; actually, there is one in each hemisphere. Its role is linked with memory, both short and long term. Licensed London taxi drivers must pass a test of their ability to drive to different locations, 'The Knowledge'. In a study of these drivers Maguire et al (2000) conducted a correlation study and concluded that this region had become enlarged as these prospective cabbies memorised and then maintained a virtual street map of London in their brains.

At normal levels of arousal, the hippocampus is dominant in handling memories. If the arousal state of our brains becomes intense the hippocampus begins to fail. In fact, faced with sustained stress the volume of the hippocampus begins to diminish (Bremner, 2006). Concurrently, the two almond shaped amygdala begin to strengthen their role in encoding these memories. Fig. 5.1 shows how the amygdala becomes increasingly dominant.

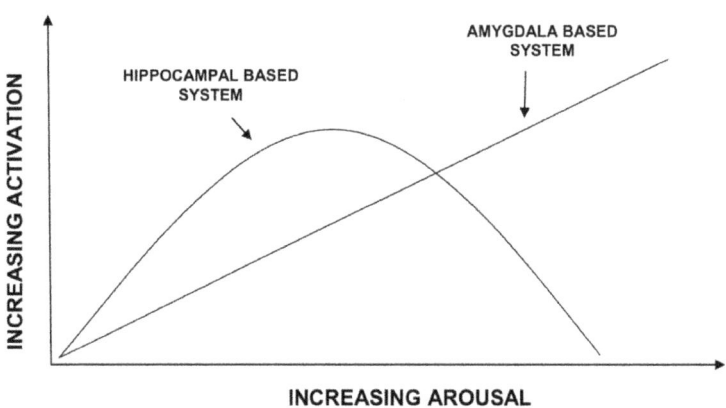

Figure 5.1 How trauma affects the way in which we encode and store memories. Lancashire Traumatic Stress Service (2013)

Apart from the lack of date stamping by the amygdala, which leaves the memories as an ever present now, they are being stored in what is the alarm centre of the brain. The amygdala are recognised for having the major role in threat processing. When we are exposed to this kind of stimuli there is a rapid transit to the amygdala. Well-connected neuronally, they initiate nerve signals supporting survival behaviours. Such threat stimuli can be perceived, and a response initiated before we even become consciously aware that anything is happening.

This mechanism is set up for survival, establishing *hypervigilance*. Consider, such a memory being encoded and memorised in this way in a theatre of war. Subsequently, the individual moves back thousands of miles to their family home. The person could well remain on *red alert* and potentially ready to react suddenly to *triggers* or *cues* that are possible reminders of the traumatic event. These could be real, similar or imaginary replays.

CONSEQUENCES

The consequences of trauma are extensive. The encoded and embedded memories have the potential to hold the individual in this state of hypervigilance. It is as if the root event remains persistently in the pending tray and has never been safely filed away. The survival mechanism that underpins the state of hypervigilance results in a tunnel vision focus on the perceived or potential threat. This will leave little bandwidth for everyday life like relationships or commitment to employment. Because it is linked to survival with adrenaline flowing persistently the affected person is likely to flare easily with outbursts of anger that are often seen by others as indiscriminate.

The initiating event or circumstances will probably leave a legacy of personal baggage, grief, loss, a lack of closure perhaps even a sense of shame. This is now overlaid with their concerns over their own behaviours and the reaction of others to their anger or erratic actions. Some trauma sufferers seek to alleviate their internal tsunami with substance abuse. The US Department of Veterans Affairs (2012) records these tragic statistics:

1. More than 2 of 10 Veterans with PTSD also have Substance Use Disorder (SUD).
- Almost 1 out of every 3 Veterans seeking treatment for SUD also has PTSD.
- The number of Veterans who smoke (nicotine) is almost double for those with PTSD (about 6 of 10) versus those without a PTSD diagnosis (3 of 10).
- In the wars in Iraq and Afghanistan, about 1 in 10 returning Veterans seen in VA have a problem with alcohol or other drugs.
- War Veterans with PTSD and alcohol problems tend to binge drink. Binge drinking is when a person drinks a lot of alcohol (4-5 drinks or more) in a short period of time (1-2 hours).

Most of us would find it challenging to maintain high levels of self-esteem when we find difficulty in applying ourselves to daily living, when our behaviours slide out from under our control and when we are haunted by past events. Our processes of self-reflection become distorted like some destructive hall of mirrors.

The amygdala are hotwired into the neural network. Renowned for their role in initiating the fight, flight or freeze response. Where that short term intention persists over time it frequently has a detrimental impact on physical health. Sleep hygiene can be sullied. The immune system can be compromised. Hypertension can be commonplace. The response intended to support our survival now impedes our ability to thrive

Unhealed trauma can lead to:

- Low sense of self worth
- Persistent fear about the future
- Co-dependency in relationships
- Fear of abandonment
- Resistance to positive change
- Tolerating abusive behaviour from others
- Craving for external validation
- Innate sense of shame
- Putting personal needs aside for others
- Not being able to tolerate conflict
- Difficulty with self-assertion and asserting boundaries
- Sycophantic

EVERYTHING CHANGES

If you have ever watched the BBC series *Peaky Blinders* (Knight 2013-2022) you will get something of the impact of trauma amongst soldiers returning from the horrors of the trench warfare of World War 1. The series depicts the flashbacks, substance abuse, incidents in the present which are rooted in previous events, and also the struggles the men have with emotionally connected relationships. Since the prevalence of confronting this pandemic of trauma, psychologists and psychiatrists have been trying to understand treat trauma, often resorting to extremes:

- utilising critical incident stress debriefing as a standard practise for helping emergency services deal with traumatic

experiences in the line of duty.
- encouraging sufferers to repeatedly relive the trauma, usually making the symptoms worse not better.
- using anti-anxiety or anti-depression drugs for years with no improvements.
- inducing diabetic comas by injecting insulin.

We constantly create a narrative in order to position ourselves in the world. This may be a constructive account which places us within a web of healthy relationships. Equally, it may be unhealthy with ourselves cast as servile pawns or even a narcissistic fable where we crown ourselves as the king or queen of our particular context. When we are confronted by trauma that narrative can undergo a seismic shift. Suddenly, the world no longer feels safe, the people that we meet can be understood as exploitative. Trust is frequently the first victim of trauma and will become a storyline in the narrative.

Confronting the toxic narrative headlong is unlikely to work as our words will become woven into that narrative of distrust. Carefully supplanting the negativity with the positive will bring changes. However, trauma drives reaction and the very mechanism of trauma is to reinforce the negative perceptions of an individual's context in order to make a response feel more insistent. It is quite common that after a traumatic experience an individual will tend to withdraw, in effect move to a place of safety. Pushing an agenda for change on an individual can create a message that something needs to be changed or fixed in us. This very message has the potential to reactivate that same trauma-based survival mechanism.

Gratitude, that recognition of goodness in our life and goodness in others and the world, can be hugely positive in offsetting trauma. Carefully managed, it is a powerful transformative tool that needs sensitive application. Wong et al (2018) conducted a fascinating study into the use of gratitude alongside other therapies. 293 adults who were receiving psychotherapy participated in a study and were randomly assigned to three groups:

1. A control group that received only psychotherapy.
2. A psychotherapy group that also did plus expressive writing focusing on expressing their deepest thoughts and feelings about stressful experiences.
3. A psychotherapy group that also did gratitude by writing letters expressing gratitude to others.

There was an evaluation made of the participants' mental health after four and twelve weeks. The group writing messages of gratitude reported better mental health than those who in the other two groups.

The authors argued that it was not positive self-expression towards oneself or others that made an impact on the participants' mental health, rather:

> It was refraining from the use of negative emotion words that explained the difference in mental health between the gratitude writing group and the expressive writing group (Wong et al., 2018).

We create our personal narratives in words. Changing, through intention, the palette of our expression from monochrome to polychrome is beneficial to all of us.

The following is a great technique for closing down the day and setting up the next one. Known as The Examen, it has been modified from a spiritual exercise developed by Ignatius of Loyola (1491-1556). Use it once and it is helpful, use it every day it is transformational. How long does it take? Up to you, anything from 5 to 30 minutes.

Step 1: Play back the day in your head, almost like a video. You can pause it, fast forward sections and even rewind.

Step 2: Highlight the good things of the day. This could include conversations, experiences, decisions, a tasty meal, an enjoyable conversation, even an act of kindness. Do not hold back, there is no audience and there will be no round of applause.

Step 3: Highlight those things that could have gone better or perhaps even the ones that you would have preferred to edit out. It might include mistakes, comments that were unkind or unnecessary, failing to care for yourself in your diet or your use of time or by getting to consumed by busyness. What might have made the day go even better?

(Care is needed here not to major on the negatives. A ratio of three positives to one negative seems to be about right).

Step 4: Make a few decisions, two or three will do. It might be something that you will do or a change of language or focus. Perhaps even plan to have a conversation with someone. Lots of possibilities but do not make them too ambitious or complicated. Quick wins are always good alongside the more sustained actions.

EMOTIONAL FREEDOM TECHNIQUE (EFT)

There is a growing recognition of the range and extent of trauma that people are trapped by. Alongside this, there is a realisation that not all talking therapies are helpful, especially those that take the traumatised person back through the very events themselves.

There is a developing interest in Eye Movement Desensitisation and Reprocessing (EMDR), which involves making rhythmic eye movements while recalling a traumatic event. It has been frequently employed to treat post-traumatic stress disorder (PTSD). An alternative to EDMR is advocated in Chapter 16, the Emotional Freedom Technique (EFT). It is straightforward to use and wide ranging in its potential application. It now comes with an increasing phalanx of supporting evidence which is taking it from being somewhat niche to becoming mainstream.

AFTERWORD

Trauma is an extremely complex area and one which should not be underplayed. Professional help should be sought as a priority in more extreme and overt situations. Simply allowing time to pass is unlikely to help. Unresolved trauma can become buried like a piece of shrapnel and impact our mental health, relationships and physical wellbeing. However, for anyone with lower levels of trauma, keeping our personal narrative positive by using a technique like The Examen and deploying EFT will be beneficial.

6

UPCYCLE

It is a cold, damp, dark February Monday morning. As you open your eyes the most attractive option is to retreat under the duvet. Instead, you get going, shower in tepid water, have a coffee, scrape the ice off the windscreen of your car and, with your breath hanging in the air, commute to work. As employment goes it is more down the OK end of the spectrum than providing stimulation and fulfilment. So, what motivated you to put yourself through running the gauntlet of discomfort to embrace a day of mediocrity. There are probably lots of different answers. Perhaps, the financial pressures of paying a mortgage or providing for a family might be the driver. Maybe mediocrity is a more attractive option than boredom or even change. Possibly work provides some level of social engagement. For some, the question is not even asked, and they are locked into a pattern that is just accepted with a level of fatalism.

Motivation is frequently mentioned by employers, teachers and even parents but seems to be frequently misunderstood. Even though a powerful cocktail of autobiography and research underscores the primacy of intrinsic motivation, the drive that comes from within, the 'go to' methods by employers and parents are so often external, (extrinsic). They are usually some variation of the 'carrot and the stick', where incentivisation is often a crude financial reward or there is the imposition of fear by an inference of job insecurity or even bullying.

There is considerable research showing that incremental financial rewards do not bring commensurate jumps in motivation. This is not a recent revelation, Deci and Ryan (1985) were looking at the way imposed, extrinsic motivation could be counterproductive. Later, Ariely et al (2005) in a study published in conjunction with US Federal Reserve Bank reached similar conclusions:

> For many tasks, introducing incentives where there previously were none or raising small incentives on the margin is likely to have a positive impact on performance. Our experiment suggests, however, that one cannot assume that introducing or raising incentives always improves performance. It now appears that beyond some threshold level, raising incentives may increase motivation to supra-optimal levels and result in perverse effects on performance. (p.21-22)

The conclusions from this research line up well with my argument. I would add a word of caution in that some of Ariely's work has faced criticism for fraud and misrepresentation of data. So here is hoping that this was one of his less controversial pieces. Further research by Irlenbusch, and Sliwka (2005) offers similar conclusions around the limitations of extrinsic motivation but lacks the drama of adverse scrutiny:

> Almost all principal-agent models imply that appropriate performance contingent monetary incentives have to be provided in order to motivate agents to exert effort. A growing number of studies, however, indicate that the provision of

monetary incentives does not necessarily lead to an increase in effort. In fact, it has been observed that incentives can even reduce the endeavours of those who were meant to become motivated. (p.1)

Our exploration is how does motivation impact our personal wellbeing. I would suggest that there are four potential issues raised by the dominant use of extrinsic motivation:

1. Financially based incentive schemes are costly; however, when there is an economic downturn retraction can have a devastating and negative effect on those involved. As the tap is turned off, feelings of anger and alienation can all too easily follow.
2. Such financial schemes, whether as direct payments or as indirect benefits such as health schemes, lead people to enter into wider commitments such as cars, loans and mortgages. If the economic climate downturns things can readily turn sour and the individual can feel trapped.
3. Extrinsic motivations can be at odds with our internal drivers. In turn, this will set up an escalating tension. If you are a person who has relationships as a significant motivator and you work in an organisation that is increasing your task rate and decreasing your contact time with people, you will feel an increasing dis-ease. I am writing this during a time where there are numbers of public sector disputes. I would suggest that whilst a living wage is needed, simply raising the percentage offer is unlikely to change situations and fulfilment at the same time.
4. Irlenbusch and Sliwka (2005), in a paper, refer to 'crowding out'. They argue that simplistic incentive schemes appear

to erode cultures of goodwill. In turn this has an impact on how people feel about themselves. Kindness and good relationships become crowded out by an ever-demanding task rate.

This is not only about the workplace. Some years ago, we moved and, in the process, lost money. We took on a house which needed a makeover. Certainly, by doing the jobs myself we gained financially but the quality of our family relationships was diminished. It was not just about time.

Motivation is arguably about our focus and also the corresponding intensity of our actions in bringing that focus to fruition. In other words, an intention needs an impetus. What is very clear is that whilst there are some basics there is a bespoke dimension to it as well.

Barratt (2020) presents a view of the brain which is less a hierarchy of structure and more a hierarchy of function:

> But we can say what is your brain's most important job. It's not rationality. Not emotion. Not imagination, or creativity, or empathy. Your brain's most important job is to control your body – to manage allostasis – by predicting energy needs before they arise so you can efficiently make worthwhile movements and survive. Your brain continually invests your energy in the hope of earning a good return, such as food, shelter, affection, or physical protection, so that you can perform nature's most vital task: passing your genes to the next generation. (p.10)

If we had no awareness of these foundational needs and took no action to secure them then we would probably die of thirst, starve, fail to take shelter and not avoid dangerous situations. We would certainly not have skin in the survival game. This entry level awareness of our basic needs and our move to get these met (motivation) has been very much part of mankind's mental toolkit since the emergence of homo sapiens. In fact, similar needs are shared with many other species.

Let's backtrack to Chapter 2 and the suggested model for mental health. A more elaborated summary of our essential needs was summarised by psychologists and psychotherapists Griffin and Tyrrell (2003). They described these as their list *primal needs*. These, the conclusion from their extensive clinical work, can be summarised as follows:

- Routinely feel safe
- Able to give and receive attention
- Have a sense of some control and influence over events in life
- Feel stretched and stimulated by life to avoid boredom
- Feel life is enjoyable
- Experience intimacy with at least one other human being
- Have a feeling of belonging to a wider community
- Have the facility to have privacy and time for personal reflection
- Have a sense of status and a reasonably defined role in life
- Have a sense of self-efficacy (personal competence)
- Have a sense of meaning and purpose

Maslow, as far back as 1943, had presented his well-known hierarchical model with physiological needs as being foundational and then topping it off with self-actualisation, his cherry on the top. This could be paraphrased as being: if you are cold, wet and hungry you are likely to be irritable, distracted and should not be trusted with anything more demanding than a tin opener. Complex tasks, which can be amongst the most fulfilling, will be relegated if lower order needs have not been sorted. An exploration of human needs has driven a wide range of literature. It underpins much the work by Seligman (2002) on Positive Psychology and probably CBT and even popularist views on motivation such as those of Al Gore's one time speech writer Pink (2009). The Tyrell and Griffin (2003) model that we are unpacking is more fluid than that of Maslow.

There is no standardised value that can be given to each of these primal needs. It is not like measuring blood pressure or sugar levels where we can take a measurement and then check it against a table of norms. We each afford them something of a personal priority and a sense of what needs to happen for them to be met in our own lives. Tyrell and Griffin's clinical practice is based on all human emotional difficulties stemming from the chronic failure to secure one or more of these primal emotional needs (Tyrell 2015).

Not only is there a lack of a standardised measurement but a number of these primal needs can be met quite differently. I worked for 17 years at University College London. On the 7th July 2005, terrorists made a number of attacks in London. Three bombs were exploded on underground trains and the fourth was detonated on a double-decker bus in Tavistock Square. Tragically, 52 people were killed and a further 700 people were injured. Two of the explosions, the bus and the underground train close to Russell Square tube station, were near where I worked. Many of my colleagues were shaken by the bombings and there was a sense of anxiety for some months afterwards in using public transport. It certainly affected me, touching on that need to feel 'routinely safe'. To avoid the underground, I bought an iconic Brompton folding bike. Over the next few years, I completed every location mentioned on a Monopoly board and many more. It seemed a good solution, though others commented about how they would not take the risk of riding a bike around Central London. Paradoxically, my solution to my need to feel safe was perceived as being terrifying by others. We will be aware of these needs but may well find our answers in very different places.

Considering some of the others:

- Feel stretched and stimulated by life to avoid boredom.
- Have a sense of self-efficacy (personal competence).
- Have a sense of meaning and purpose.

Then people can meet these needs in many different ways. Extending oneself through study or work could come through learning a new language, climbing Kilimanjaro or even buying a dog. One person may develop a sense of self-efficacy through playing the piano, another through becoming a surgeon and yet another by playing sport. Meaning and purpose could come through belonging to a religious organisation, supporting cancer research, being part of a team or planting out a garden.

There are no easy answers to finding a pathway through to understanding our personal motivations and how we meet these in order to discover and maintain personal fulfilment. A friend has just started a YouTube Channel. Titled *Confessions of a Headmaster* (Holloway 2023) there was always going to some viewers being disappointed at the lack/absence of salacious content. He suggests that each of us have two particularly important days in our lives; firstly, the date that we are born and secondly the day that we find out why we were born. That connects beautifully with the trajectory of this chapter. My friend's assertion has certainly made me pause and think. Perhaps we give excessive weighting to the 'how' of our lives and scant regard to the 'why'.

Pink (2009), following a career as a political speech writer, investigated motivation. He has manged to distil a great deal of the thinking around motivation and in particular those deeper life root areas into three dimensions:

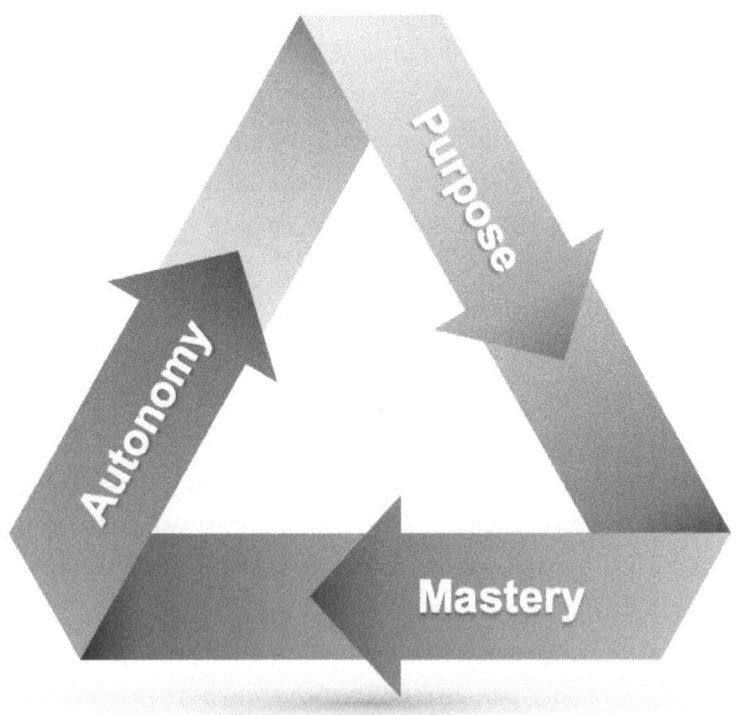

Fig. 6.1 Three dimensions of motivation

Pink argues for motivation operating in a deep and meaningful way in each of us and points to the need needs to feel some level of autonomy. There is usually some level of compromise as we work and share with those around us. However, if we feel that we are trapped and have no freedom to contribute or time to walk our own path at times we will feel stressed. The advice given to people being tortured was to hold back their scream for even a few seconds to reduce the imposition of victim status by their tormentors. Perhaps not the most pleasant illustration but it makes a point. I was a secondary school head for 14 years. A major preoccupation was challenging students not to wear trainers, do their top button up and tuck their shirt in! Such infringements were an almost inevitable consequence of having a uniform with its impact on adolescent autonomy.

Moving on and perhaps reaching for some more creative demonstrations of autonomy. Book tickets for a concert by an artist of your choice, wear odd socks, write with a fountain pen, go to Skegness on your holidays, become a vegetarian, drive a Land Rover and park it next to a hybrid or carve spoons with an axe. These are relatively small potatoes, though holidaying in Skegness might require courage. However, what about changing your job or your career with associated retraining or study for a degree if that was not open to you when you were younger.

What are you good at? That is a very different question for saying how good are you at something? Each of us needs to have a sense of mastery or self-efficacy, that is an ability to perform in an area in a way that gives us a sense of achievement. This could be the short-term completion of a task or project; equally it could be embedded in a hard-won skill. The list is endless; however, a lack of some area of accomplishment and a lack of a forum for its performance will diminish us.

Self-efficacy can be demonstrated by an action like playing an instrument or completing a task and is quite different from self-esteem. The latter is about feelings and is usually serviced by the residual messages that we have been given by others. Many of us live our lives with defining messages echoing around our heads: 'You're useless', ' You're not musical', ' You're stupid', or even more muted versions such as 'You've not done badly considering' or 'You've done better than I expected'. I have been hearing impaired nearly all my life. When I was thirteen my performance dropped significantly over a single term, top of the class to the bottom in ten weeks. I simply could not hear what was going on and I was even punished when I asked another pupil what had been said. I was booked in for a medical. To this day I remember the doctor telling me mother that she had done well to get me this far but not to expect much more. A write-off at thirteen? Fortunately, I ignored the diagnosis, but it still caused me to question my right to succeed. My self-esteem was severely dented and it took a lot of mental panel beating to get the dents out.

Purpose is probably even more individualistic. However, the personal erosion we feel is seldom caused by not having the right purpose but rather a lack of purpose. To feel that you are an orphan in an infinite universe is dispiriting. There are levels of purpose ranging from being part of a team that is developing something through to articulating our spiritual engagement and finding where we are comfortable in our skin and at home in the cosmos.

Pink does not offer definitive advice on where we might position ourselves in these categories. There is work to do in each of these three areas. It may take several years to bottom them out. To leave them unresolved will leave us stressed as we struggle with their deficit.

For several generations my family reared turkeys in Norfolk. I remember my mother telling me that they lived in a manor house with a ballroom. My expectations took a sharp downturn when she added that that was where they kept the turkeys. A legacy of family wisdom from that time was that it is always unwise to stuff a live turkey; an extended description is not really needed here and the image will probably haunt your dreams. It is a great metaphor though for the limited way motivation is commonly approached. We are forced into roles and performance by motivational practices that are crude and archaic. We all too frequently become victims of coercion and our autonomy, purpose and mastery are stripped back leaving us in a personal shadowland.

7

HOW LOW CAN YOU GET?

> How will we better contain depression? Expect no magic pill. One lesson learned from treating chronic pain is that it is tough to override responses that are hardwired into the body and the mind. Instead, we must follow the economy of mood where it leads, attending to the sources that brings so many into low mood states – think routines that feature too much work and too little sleep. We need broader mood literacy and an awareness of tools that interrupt low mood states before they morph into longer more severe ones. These tools include altering how we think the events around us, our relationships, and conditions in our body.
>
> (Rottenberg, 2014, p. 32)

In the 1950s, my father worked as an engineer for a Stafford-based grinding wheel company. He regularly visited a factory in Leeds that made asbestos-based building products such as roofing materials and downpipes. Several streets from the factory, he saw children having 'snowball fights' with toxic asbestos waste that was just blowing around the streets like malignant tumbleweed. The actual conditions in the factory must have been terminal. Over the years we have recognised an ever-increasing roll of occupational-based diseases. These have included pneumoconiosis for miners who repeatedly inhaled coal dust, or even mercury poisoning experienced by Victorian hatters, an occupation immortalised by Lewis Carroll.

Anxiety and depression are extremely widespread in society. Perhaps it is time to add these to the roll of occupation-related diseases? Though that is probably not feasible as our heads are a 'one stop shop'. Your employment might be adversely affecting the quality of our mental health. However, your head is also the receptacle for everything else that is going on around you and is topped up with relationship breakdown, isolation, debt, health concerns, bullying, personal identity as well as global impositions like climate change, the war in Ukraine and pandemics. So, perhaps anxiety and depression are the occupational disease of just living. However, are they inevitable?

The World Health Organisation (WHO) (2021) and Seligman (1988) both suggested that people born since 1945 are ten times more likely to suffer from depression than those born before this date. This is startling, particularly when you consider that many of those born before 1945 went through the World Wars and suffered associated deprivation. In that same article, the WHO concluded that depression is a frontrunner in the cause of disability worldwide. This is massively significant and probably what many people connect with when they say they have mental health issues.

WHAT IT IS AND WHAT IT DOES

Robert had been the lead trainer in a management consultancy firm and had worked for them for five years. His contribution to the organisation was seen as being significant and positive. Unexpectedly, a series of issues cascaded to generate high levels of personal stress. He had challenged the unacceptable performance of one of the team and it had rapidly escalated into an unpleasant stand-off as she was signed off with stress. Sadly, the lady had also suffered a miscarriage. She submitted a complaint that accused Robert of bullying behaviour and that this had been a contributory cause of the miscarriage. Compassionate by nature, this affected Robert deeply. Meanwhile the company was undertaking major restructuring which left the workforce feeling uncertain and insecure. At a personal level, Robert was also facing anxiety. His father, who suffered from Parkinson's Disease, was becoming increasingly infirm and unable to maintain independent living. When he snatched some less-pressured moments for himself, he felt guilty about his increasing detachment from his wife and his teenage children. Dark clouds had suddenly appeared in what had been a clear blue sky.

He was aware that he was being affected by these events: he was exhausted; simple tasks were beginning to feel insurmountable; he suffered from mood swings. As his confidence ebbed away, hope was becoming a distant horizon and increasingly anger and criticism were becoming personal motifs. Normally gregarious, he was now starting to detach himself from people and realised that he was becoming self-absorbed and ruminating on his problems. Whilst he was not particularly keen on hobbies, he did enjoy walking his dog and eating out. A moment's reflection revealed a somewhat neglected dog and a growing number of unmemorable meals.

Feeling less than his best, Robert had sought medical advice. His GP assured him that there was no underlying pathology such as heart disease or thyroid problems. He diagnosed Robert as being depressed and suggested that he took time off work for at least a month and that he should start a course of anti- depressants. These were not his solutions of choice. Being absent from work for a month seemed to be the stuff of fantasy. He decided not to take the anti-depressants after an internet search about their potential side effects. There seemed to be some evidence that they could impair his core role as a decision-maker (Crockett *et al*, 2015).

Seamlessly, anxiety had morphed into depression.

Many people who are depressed just keep going and many around them are not even aware of their plight. The impact on the individual's functioning will require more effort and determination to try to keep their perceived normality on track. This can be misleading. Flintham (2003) in research on secondary headteachers recorded this comment by one person that he interviewed:

> I was very good at hiding it. Other heads and my staff didn't know the extent of my angst until I lost it through a panic attack at a heads' meeting. I went long-term sick and had to retire early on health grounds. I've cut myself off from education. I've never been back to my school and at first, I couldn't even face the people I'd worked with if I met them elsewhere. I don't work at all now. (p. 8)

THE STRUCTURE OF DEPRESSION

Robert had become overwhelmed by challenging circumstances, but context was not the total explanation. Problems and issues that we have to deal with can have an attached emotional tag. A significant dispute with a colleague might not leave us professionally detached. Just institute a process and appoint a replacement; job done. Situations like this can create anxiety and rumination. In this example, the situation was exacerbated by the allegations that had been made by the employee. Similarly,

Daniel in an earlier chapter had become mired in toxicity and circumstances.

Such emotional tags will usually trigger a stress state and in turn this will change our style of thinking. The brain will also try to bring such emotional arousal to a completion. We do not like unresolved situations. If we do not achieve this during the day then it will end up in the inbox of our nocturnal downtime called Rapid Eye Movement (REM) sleep. More of this later.

Depressed people will often use language which reflects their retreat into a tight inner focus and place themselves very much in the centre. Their statements will become increasingly black and white or what is often typified as 'all-or-nothing thinking'. A depressed person will tend to talk in terms of the situation 'as always being like this' or a potential resolution as being 'the only alternative'. The latter somehow feels like an oxymoron but people still use the expression. They will often perceive good things as temporary and random whilst bad things are understood as being permanent and deserved. If you remember the discussion of the fight-or-flight response, it was argued that stress inhibits alternatives in order to facilitate a rapid response to an immediate and non-deferrable threat. This begins to explain many of the hallmarks of depression: the blindness to consider the needs of others, the failure to engage with tasks, the disregard of the longer term and the impact of the adrenaline rush and the activation of the amygdala (brain's alarm centres) potentially manifesting as anger.

Additionally, the world keeps turning. Work-related and personal decisions must still be made. These are now being made with an impaired thinking process. If these new problems cannot be resolved then there will be further anxiety and rumination and so the depression wheel keeps turning. Robert found himself facing a number of pressing issues to which there were no easy answers. Rittell and Webber (1973) formalised the description of these kind of problems as being 'wicked'. These are problems which often lack clear definition and where the solution is pragmatic rather than absolute. However, what is clear is that these kinds of problems are portable and soon become constant companions.

Such problems have attached unclosed emotional loops. These unresolved loops become the substance of our dreams as the brain creates scenarios and metaphorically acts these out in an attempt to close these loops. For example, anxiety caused by someone making critical comments about you could manifest in a dream where you are mugged and beaten up. Dreams occur during the REM period of our sleep; this process is our emotional launderette. The following chapter, *Living the dream,* describes sleep as not only busy but also vitally important to our wellbeing and vital in combating depression. Dreaming is hard work.

If our dreaming is not managing to close these emotional loops then we will sow the seeds of depression in the tilth of pessimistic and narrowed patterns of language. Attempts to resolve these demand that more and more time is spent in REM sleep, and this also begins to appear earlier in the sleep cycle. A depressed person does up to three times as much dreaming in the REM state that a non-depressed person does. Further, in a person who is not depressed, REM sleep cuts in some 90 minutes after falling asleep, whereas in a depressed person it can start as quickly as three minutes after falling asleep.

When we engage in REM sleep, serotonin is depleted. Serotonin (there are actually quite a few types) serves a number of functions, including sponsoring our physical motivation.

During REM sleep it helps suppress muscle movement; we become almost paralysed to ensure that our dreams remain metaphorical and are not acted out in a potentially dangerous manner. With this depletion of serotonin, we wake tired and find we really are not set up to get going physically. Serotonin is a neurotransmitter with a role which also includes generating feelings of fulfilment or completion. Imagine pushing your chair back after a satisfying meal feeling replete; that is very much the sort of feeling it generates. If, however, it has been depleted from an excess of REM sleep, we are also more likely to feel empty, aimless and purposeless. A lack of serotonin does not cause depression, but rather depression leads to its depletion. We have different cycles of sleep and if REM sleep is excessive then, Slow-wave Sleep is minimised and so refreshment and healing can be inhibited as well. A significant part of the package of depression is over-dreaming. It is not uncommon for people experiencing depression to wake up regularly just to gain respite from the spinning and unresolved dreaming in the REM phase.

RESET

Depression should never be trivialised, either in ourselves or in others. The fact that it is such a prevalent mental health issue makes it no less serious and it can easily become the gateway to incapacity and even self-harm. If you suspect you are depressed or that a colleague or friend is treading this well-worn path, then medical advice should be sought or strongly advocated. If, as you are reading this, you are already taking prescription medication for anxiety or depression, please do not stop taking it or alter the dosage without discussing this with your doctor. Advice or strategy in this chapter – or indeed, in the book as a whole – can be used in tandem with medical intervention.

The above is very much a 'flypast' of the subject of depression. This evidence- based perspective of both explanatory style and the role of over-dreaming has been of benefit to many people in moving on from the debilitating effects of depression. A much more extensive and indeed practical consideration is given in *How to lift depression...fast* (Griffin and Tyrell, 2014a):

1. *Understand how depression works, then if we can see it for what it is, we can intercept the behaviours that are driving the cycle. Once understood and viewed as something that can be resolved and that our situation can be changed, a light will begin to appear at the end of the tunnel: hope. Development of these insights is best done routinely outside of a depressive episode so that you have tools which are both preventative and curative at your disposal – but it is never too late to use them. The following strategies will certainly be effective in pulling us out of the quagmire of depression and they are also useful to prevent us bogging down in the first place. Audit your life on a weekly basis and really commit to this with no downtime. (A way of auditing our thinking is outlined in Chapter 20).*
2. *Secure good sleeping patterns so that the toll of over-dreaming is avoided or minimised. This will significantly reduce the fatigue and the joint and muscle pains that are so often the hallmarks of depression.*
3. *It is useful to 'listen in' to our conversations, both internal and external. Are our stories becoming pessimistic? Is our language increasingly peppered with 'all-or-nothing phrases' that give away our restricted and damaging thinking? Does our self-talk condemn us? It would be useful to notice whether we speak to others in an uninterested,*

angry or irritated fashion. Are we taken up with too much meaning-making and catastrophisation? We can check and/or explore our language and phraseology and how to reframe our narrative (Chapter 11).

4. *One of the single most successful strategies for resetting depression is mindfulness (Chapter 17). It has been estimated that we exist 'in the moment' for a mere two hours during the time that we are formally awake. The remainder of the time, we try to understand past events or we move into an inappropriate prophetic mode as we try to anticipate the future. Mindfulness brings us back to the present and reduces rumination. It is like pulling up in a layby with an overheated engine and changing into neutral and letting the engine idle and cool down. Routinely practising mindfulness has an enduring effect by helping us view problems in a less intense and pressing manner. When I work with depressed or anxious clients, this (now widely known) technique is welcomed as being a positive strategy. In many cases, however, the benefits are negated if the client is not practising it on a daily basis. A two-day trial will change little. It has sometimes been treated with indifference and even greeted with cynicism. Intermittent use is the equivalent of the diabetic leaving their insulin in the medicine cabinet. Perhaps singing 'Let It Go' from Disney's Frozen (2013) should be mandatory (This should probably only be done in tightly prescribed situations to avoid damaging personal credibility!).*

5. *Ensure that you make time for pleasure, fun or social activity. It is important that this is something that appeals to you and is not an activity which someone else feels that you should do. Sometimes this might require making*

an effort and moving out of your temporary, depressed, discomfort zone.
6. When we are depressed, we become self-absorbed and almost anything that expands our interpersonal horizons will be beneficial. The positive psychologist Martin Seligman (2008) suggests setting up a 'gratitude visit'. You are asked to think of someone who has made a significant positive contribution to your life but is unaware of the fact. Seligman suggests writing down a 300-word testimonial and then making an appointment to go and see them but not to declare the intended purpose of your visit. Seligman admits that the meeting will be emotional but in a good way. This is an interesting technique, but probably it would not be appropriate for someone who was feeling at a particularly low point.
7. Healthy diet and exercise will always help our general health. Exercise has been recognised as being particularly beneficial (Craft and Perna, 2004). If you have not exercised for a long time or are concerned about the effects of exercise has on your body or health, ask your GP about exercise on prescription. Many GP surgeries across the country prescribe exercise as a treatment for a range of conditions, including depression.
8. Spend time with people who are not depressed. They do not need to be stand-up comedians, though some level of positivity on their part will certainly be beneficial. Some 15 years ago I experienced a significant bout of depression. I was off work and I was invited round for coffee by a friend in similar circumstances. In the three weeks that he had been off work, he had become a leading expert on depression. What he did not know about possible medication and

counselling really was not worth knowing or so he told me. I left determined to avoid him and find more uplifting company. Now, all these years on, he is still being treated for depression, and sadly he has developed 'depression as lifestyle'. I will come clean; I went and spent a week with a friend, camping and making a chair using a pole lathe. This friend was just this side of hilarious. You cannot get an experience like this on the NHS, but it did reinforce the fact that the opposite of depression is not happiness but peace!

9. *Counselling, one of the talking therapies. This can be useful but a depressed person should avoid psychodynamic counsellors who seek to explore the past. If you are depressed then a future-focused therapy, rather than one which supports rumination about the past, will win the day. Interestingly, in America some psychodynamic counsellors have been sued by clients who have come to them with depression and found themselves to be in a worse state than when they started their therapy (Elliott and Griffin, 2002).*

AFTERWORD

Life events, including those from our professional and personal arenas, can be seen to trigger depression. Depression is not, however, caused by what happens to us; it is about how we respond and make sense of these events. This understanding of how depression is constructed and ultimately treated has been developed by Griffin and Tyrell:

> The important thing is to know how depression is manufactured in the brain. Once you understand that, you can correct

the maladaptive cycle incredibly fast. For 40 years it's been known that depressed people have excessive REM sleep. They dream far more than healthy people. What we realised – and proved – is that the negative introspection, or ruminations, that depressed people engage in actually causes the excessive dreaming. So, depression is being generated on a 24-hour cycle and we can make a difference within 24 hours to how a person feels. (2014b, p. 6)

8

LIVING THE DREAM

> The machinery is always going. Even when you are asleep.
>
> (Andy Warhol)

It had been one of those days; the intentions of the morning had given way to the frustrations of the afternoon. The unexpected had progressively eclipsed the 'to-do list'. Arriving home at 7.30 p.m, you ate a meal with no recollection of what you had eaten. Two hours were spent catching up with unfinished work from the day. Finally, exhausted, you managed to get into bed, sliding between freshly laundered sheets, echoing Quasimodo's cry of 'Sanctuary'. Nothing could be further from the truth. This is where a session of serious work is about to begin. If sleep does not progress in a defined pattern, there will be serious consequences in terms of wellbeing and personal efficacy. Disturbed sleep is not simply about feeling tired at the start of the following day, it is about leaving life events in untidy stacks in our heads and leaving emotional loops unresolved.

THE INNER GAME OF SLEEP

Most of us spend approximately one third of our lives sleeping, or at least trying to sleep. A simple survey will soon show that many people have little idea of what is happening beyond a having a somewhat vague belief that a good night's sleep is desirable. Robotham, Chakkalackal and Cyhlarova (2011) make the argument for sleep as a core human activity:

> Sleep affects our ability to use language, sustain attention, understand what we are reading and summarise what we are hearing. If we compromise on our sleep, we compromise on our performance, our mood and our interpersonal relationships. (p. 13)

Good sleep is held to have a series of five stages, and in turn these groupings occur some four or five times each night, with each cycle taking around 90 minutes. The first stage is light sleep, almost an interface between being awake and being asleep. This is the stage where we can get those strange twitches called hypnic jerks. A few minutes later we move into Stage 2, not dissimilar to Stage 1 but that bit deeper with muscles relaxing, eye movement stopping and a slowing of heart and breathing rates. This stage accounts for nearly 50% of human sleep but it is still fairly shallow and someone woken at this point could well deny that they have even been asleep.

Stages 3 and 4 are normally grouped together and the distinction between them is technical and is linked to the proportion of different brain waves. This stage is often referred to as slow-wave sleep. This type of sleep is refreshing, and waking someone from this stage will often result in the sleeper feeling disorientated and they will appear only semi coherent. Importantly, this is where what has been learnt during the day is processed and incorporated into our memories. It is in some ways like saving a document or spreadsheet to the hard drive.

The final stage of each cycle, if all is going to plan, is rapid eye movement (REM) sleep. This takes its name from the discernible eye movements that can be seen under the closed eyelids. The breathing rate rises, as does the heart rate. Concurrently, the major muscle groups become paralysed so that we cannot move our arms and legs.

It is during REM sleep that we begin to dream. Mystery still surrounds the role of dreaming. Some contend that important emotional processing is taking place, whilst others seem to suggest that they are little more than a device to keep the brain occupied so that the sleeper does not wake up (Solms, 2000). In the following chapter, the argument is made that, whilst there is still a great deal to be discovered about REM sleep, its role is considerably more important than being a psychological Netflix.

These five stages, which are iterative, are regulated by a mechanism called a circadian timer working in tandem with the sleep homeostat. The latter is a regulator that secures adequate amounts of sleep and can implement a payback process if we have built up a sleep debt through not being able to get sufficient sleep over the preceding period. This complex feedback mechanism is controlled by periods of light and darkness. The way these two interact is shown in Fig. 8.1 below:

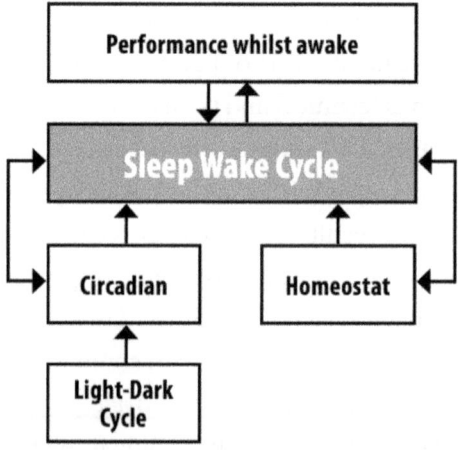

Figure 8.1 *Sleep homeostat and circadian timer (Dijk, 2010, in Robotham , Chakkalackal and Cyhlarova 2011, p. 17)* 87

Too much detail? However, it does give an indication that this watch-like mechanism is susceptible to being thrown out of kilter.

A prolonged period of stress or worry can also affect our ability to sleep. In a sample of roughly 20,000 young adults, lack of sufficient sleep was linked to psychological distress.
Robotham , Chakkalackal and Cyhlarova (2011, p. 31)

SLEEP WALKING

Sleepio is an organisation exploring sleep patterns and it also providing advice to help people improve the quality of their sleep. They also conduct regular surveys of sleeping habits in the UK. The data used below is taken from their 2011 and 2012 surveys. Their findings provide insights as to how sleep empowers performance and its lack will cause us to operate below par.

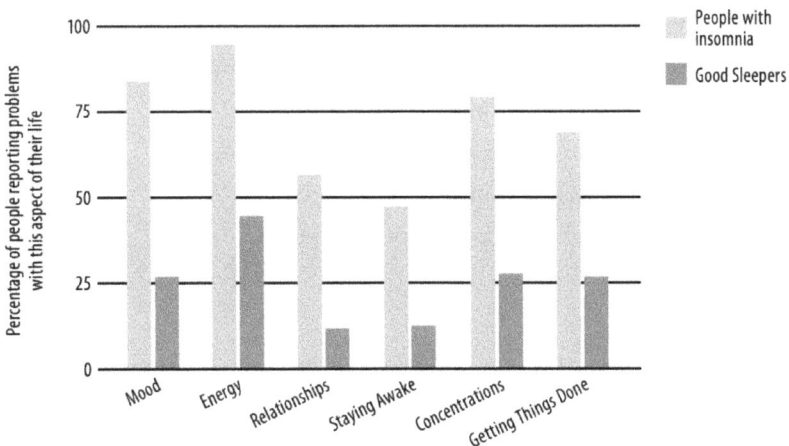

Graph 8.1 *The Negative impact of poor sleep on daily life (Robotham , Chakkalackal and Cyhlarova, 2011, p. 31)*

The data from the survey, presented here as a graph, is unequivocal in showing that the effects of poor sleep have a major impact on our daily activities. When a comparison is made between good sleepers and their sleep deprived counterparts, many in the latter group have reported having four times as many relationship difficulties. The results also show that low mood increases with poor sleep patterns, as does an increased susceptibility to depression.

Insomniac respondents reported issues around reduced concentration and poor energy levels. They found difficulty in 'getting things done' and staying awake.

The latter would certainly affect performance at work. However, in turn a failure to cope with tasks effectively will inevitably increase anxiety and (dis)stress.

The survey of the following year (2012) displayed similar trends. Poor sleepers in comparison with those with good sleep patterns are:

- seven times more likely to feel helpless;
- five times more likely to feel alone;
- three times more likely to struggle to concentrate;
- twice as likely to suffer from fatigue;
- twice as likely to have relationship problems;
- twice as likely to suffer low mood;
- twice as likely to be unproductive.

(Sleepio, 2012, p. 3)

The extension of these findings to include feelings around helplessness and a perception of being isolated should be of concern to all of us.

The wild card in terms of sleep disturbance has been the Covid 19 Pandemic, possibly linked to the associated psychological distress. The effects of this in the longer term are not clear at the time of writing.

> Altered sleep patterns and specific sleep-related symptoms are common in the general population during the pandemic lockdown. These are mainly associated with mental health impact, self-isolation, suspected COVID-19 infection and ongoing symptoms. The potential consequences of the lockdown on sleep should not be overlooked, as they can have an impact on the future wellbeing of society. Sleep issues may be addressed early with appropriate guidance and/or counselling to avoid the longer-term impact of these on a public health scale.
>
> (Perez- Carbonell et al 2020, p. 173)

DREAMS ARE MADE OF THIS

Securing a good night's sleep should be high on all of our personal agendas. The challenging question is: how much sleep do we need? There is no definitive answer to this question. A new-born baby may sleep for 18 hours a day whilst someone in middle age may manage with as little as five hours each night. The structure of sleep may vary with young people who record a greater incidence of REM sleep. This is probably linked to brain maturation. REM sleep is also associated with the plasticity of neuronal networks, which could help with the acquisition of new skills.

Taking a slight detour, Dijk and Winsky-Sommerer (2012) noted that during adolescence sleep becomes shallower and shifts to later hours. They also argued that:

The frontal lobe – responsible for executive functions such as planning and inhibiting inappropriate behaviour – shows a marked fall in synapse density as the result of neuronal pruning. Teenagers are not just being lazy when they don't want to get out of bed. Their adolescent biology may also prefer an adjustment of school hours.

There is good evidence that young people don't get enough sleep. When they live on an 8-hour sleep schedule they remain sleepy, and much more so than older people on the same schedule. If young adults are forced to stay in bed in darkness for 16 hours a day they initially sleep for as long as 12 hours. However, after several days they level off to just under 9 hours, showing that they were paying off a sleep debt. (2012, p. 3)

Whilst it is difficult to be precise about the amount of sleep that we need, it is indisputable that we all need good quality sleep if we are to remain well and to function at a high level. There are many reasons why people suffer from insomnia and it is advisable to seek medical advice if you are not sleeping on a regular basis. What follows is general advice that will help you sleep well:

1. **Relax before going to bed.** Take time for a pre-sleep ritual to break the link between your daytime activity and bedtime. You might try some mindfulness, reading or a shower.
2. **Avoid caffeine.** Coffee, tea, and hot chocolate generally contain the stimulant caffeine.
3. **Note anything on your mind.** If there is something that you are thinking about, or something that you need to remember, write it down in a notebook. The latter is better

than scraps of paper, which can be lost, and better than a smartphone, which should not be in the bedroom anyway!
4. **Limit alcohol consumption.** Alcoholic drinks may help you to fall asleep, but as your body clears the alcohol from your system, you are likely to wake up. It can also cause disturbing dreams, sweating and headaches. Drinking one glass of water for every unit of alcohol consumed will help but then you begin to run into problems associated with number 6!
5. **Your bed is for sleeping in.** Your mind attaches significance to particular locations. It is helpful to build an expectation that this is the place where sleep happens. It is useful to avoid TV, digital devices, intense discussions and even eating when you are in bed.
6. **No drinks after 8.00.** This can seem harsh but if you wish to avoid trips to the 'loo' during the night then this is sound advice unless there are medical reasons why you should continue with your fluid intake.
7. **Eat for sleep.** Avoid eating a large meal just before bedtime and conversely do not go to bed hungry. Sleep-supportive snacks include milk, tuna, almonds, eggs, peaches, oats, asparagus, potatoes and bananas.
8. **Exercise at the right time.** Regular exercise can relieve stress and encourage sleep. However, exercising in the latter part of the evening to the extent that your blood is pumping will probably stimulate you too much.
9. **Create the right environment.** Your bedroom should be a quiet pace with subdued lighting and a temperature around 20-22 degrees Celsius. If you read, it is better to have a point source of light rather than raising the overall level of lighting in the room.

10. **Power nap.** There are many advocates of the daytime power nap and in some countries some level of sleep during the day is part of the culture. However, if you routinely fall asleep in the evening then the support act will eclipse the star attraction.

This chapter, *Living the dream*, has explored the importance of sleep in terms of our performance. It connects with the chapter on depression *Chapter 7, How low can you get?* And *Chapter 14, Strike a happy medium'*, also has advice on the impact of digital devices and considers their adverse effect on our sleep.

Sometimes, we are own worst enemies by not making adequate preparations for this vital part of our lives. After all, if we spend one-third of our lives sleeping or attempting to sleep, let us at least take such a vital process seriously.

9

BREAKING BAD

Several years ago, I mentioned to friends that I was going to make my own gin. The project was not greeted with the enthusiasm that I was expecting. Some questioned the legality of running a still. I explained that I had worked that one through. A number of others suggested that my gin might be toxic and cause blindness. I countered this with the assurance that I had originally studied chemistry and that it would be safe. At this point, the universal response was, 'Had I seen the TV series *Breaking Bad*?' (Gilligan 2008 – 2013). The story line of the series follows the misadventures of Walter White, a dispirited high school teacher with lung cancer. He makes the transition from teaching to producing the illegal recreational drug, crystal meth. I did not see the comparison as a compliment.

Moving on. The human body is an intriguing chemical factory and like all complex systems is prone to malfunction. Keeping it running and resolving its glitches is a massive commercial / industrial enterprise Between 2021-2022 it had a global value put at 1.48 trillion dollars (Mikulic 2023). Most of us have benefitted from its innovations and products, in fact, many of us might not be reading this without taking, for example, antibiotics. Despite its huge positive impact on the human race, the industry as a whole should not be viewed as altogether benign or altruistic.

In the same way that flies swarm near rotting meat, so commercial enterprises can be corrupted by the eye wateringly large revenues. There are numerous examples where errors in this industry have had catastrophic consequences. Consider the case of the anti-cholesterol drug, Cerivastatin, made by the German pharmaceutical company Bayer. It was marketed from 1997 and withdrawn in 2001. There have been multimillion dollar claims filed against Bayer after it was withdrawn and initially linked to 100 deaths. *The Lancet* (2003) recorded this fascinating ethical deviation by Bayer as these claims came to trial:-

> The first case came to trial in Corpus Christi, Texas, last week, and Bayer was immediately in deep water in court. The company had sent a letter to over 2000 local residents, reminding them that it employs nearly 2000 people in Texas and contributes about US$185 million to the state's economy in payroll, taxes, and support of local groups. (p. 793)

This quotation takes the ethical issues beyond issues around the original drug trials. So, clearly sections of the pharmaceutical industry are not above reproach.

The eclipse of the value of service to humanity by commercial practice was outed by Henry Gadsden. Thirty years ago, Gadsden was the CEO of the pharmaceutical giant Merck, in an interview with Fortune magazine he said that he wanted Merck 'to be more like chewing gum maker Wrigley's' (Barratt 2006, p. 93). He was overt in declaring that his dream was to sell prescription drugs to healthy people and provide a universal market for Merck. A strangely similar trajectory of travel to that of the Colombian drug cartels.

As a postscript, it is intriguing that the routinely cited Gadsden quotation is so difficult to reference. I have used it a number of times in the last ten years or so and I have seldom accessed it the same way. It is a seminal quotation on the practices of big pharma and yet it shares much with the Cheshire cat's smile.

Journalists Moynihan and Cassels (2006) take Gadsden's aspiration as their starting point. They argue that pharmaceutical companies are engaged in widening the boundaries that define illness and that by doing this they can increase their potential market:

> Mild problems are painted as a serious disease, so shyness becomes a sign of social anxiety disorder and pre-menstrual tension, a mental illness called pre-menstrual dysphoric disorder. Everyday sexual difficulties are seen as sexual dysfunctions, the natural change of life is a disease of hormone deficiency called the menopause, and distracted office workers now have adult ADD. Just being at 'risk of an illness' has now become a 'disease' in its own right, so healthy middle-aged women now have a silent bone disease called osteoporosis and fit middle-aged men a lifelong condition called high cholesterol. (p.vx)

It is suggested that some care is needed here. The gist of their argument is made in a clear fashion. However, their journalistic zeal should not be allowed to cloud the real benefits that statins taken to reduce cholesterol have brought or the very real relief that many women have enjoyed as a result of taking HRT.

Moynihan and Cassels go on to argue that the relationship between pharmaceutical companies and doctors is somewhat incestuous. They report that 90% of people who sit on clinical guidelines committees have conflicts of interest because of financial ties to pharmaceutical companies. These are the committees that consider the ethical issue around clinical trials. Stop for a moment and consider who else would be on those committees but clinicians. However, it is the bias creating financial ties that could be problematical.

This fusion surfaces elsewhere. Originating in the USA is an influential publication, the *Diagnostic and Statistical Manual* (DSM). In its various iterations the authors categorise mental health issues and seek to capture as many as they can. However, it is important to understand that not all of the claims made for it being a comprehensive collection stack up. Started in 1952, it listed 106 mental disorders. Homosexuality was only removed from the manual in 1974. DSM-5 (2013) now lists more than 250 disorders. In its last format, they sought entries from the general public. Pickersgill (2013) a strong critic of this later version of DSM (DSM-5), identifies a trend:

> In some senses, there is nothing especially novel about the debates noted above: critics have long attacked the validity and reliability of the DSM, and indeed the wider kinds of medicalisation it is often deemed to promote. Relating to this are criticisms of the role of drugs for mental health conditions. The pharmaceutical industry can be regarded as what Jutel calls an 'engine of diagnosis', which helps to power changes to the APA nosology and then becomes further embroiled in the processes of medicalisation that help to support 'pharmaceuticalisation'. (p. 3)

At the heart of Pickersgill's critique is the concern that if you can label something as a pathology or disease, then in turn you have a platform from which to prescribe medication(s).

In many ways this was Gadsden's dream come true. In the revision of the DSM to its fifth version 67% (18/27) of the committee had direct links to pharmaceutical companies (*Nursing Time*s 2013). Is this simply too many with such links to maintain objectivity?

Depression is debilitating, widespread and it haemorrhages hope. The revenue on its treatment is massive with £35 million in April 2020 being spent by the NHS alone (Robinson 2021). The use of such prescription medications to treat depression and anxiety is far from simple. Further, the commercial opportunities presented by such treatments could muddy the waters as an inappropriate fusion between science and marketing develops.

There are many studies around the effectiveness of antidepressant medications. One of the more accessible is the research of Kirsch (2014). In essence, antidepressants are prescribed to resolve a chemical imbalance in the brain. Many that are currently prescribed are classed as Selective Serotonin Reuptake inhibitors (SSRIs). These include Zoloft and Prozac. It is argued that the levels of the neurotransmitter, serotonin, are depleted in the brains of people suffering depression and so conserving it by definition must be good. Kirsch (2014) noted that in France, Tianeptine is prescribed for depression. This is a medication that actually depletes serotonin, a so called Selective Setatonin Reuptake Enhancer (SSRE). The outcomes from the diametrically opposite drugs were identical. This makes no sense at all. It is probably safest to quote directly from Kirsch himself:

> Antidepressants are supposed to work by fixing a chemical imbalance, specifically, a lack of serotonin in the brain. Indeed, their supposed effectiveness is the primary evidence for the

chemical imbalance theory. But analyses of the published data and the unpublished data that were hidden by drug companies reveals that most (if not all) of the benefits are due to the placebo effect. Some antidepressants increase serotonin levels, some decrease it, and some have no effect at all on serotonin. Nevertheless, they all show the same therapeutic benefit. Even the small statistical difference between antidepressants and placebos may be an enhanced placebo effect, due to the fact that most patients and doctors in clinical trials successfully break blind. The serotonin theory is as close as any theory in the history of science to having been proved wrong. Instead of curing depression, popular antidepressants may induce a biological vulnerability making people more likely to become depressed in the future. (2014, p. 1)

(When patients break blind it means that they have guessed that they are on a medication rather than a placebo or sugar pill. To counter this 'active placebos' have been developed which mimic the potential side-effects but do not have any therapeutic value.)

Surely, if the medication works even at the level of a placebo then that might be some justification for their use. However, anti-depressants are powerful and they are far from harmless. The use of SSRIs for people under the age of 24 actually doubles the risk of suicide (FDA 2004).

This book is not advocating throwing your medicinal crutches away and shouting 'It's a miracle'. Starting or stopping any medication, or changing the dose, should only be undertaken on the advice of a qualified medical practitioner. The argument here, is to suggest exploring alternatives to an exclusive reliance on medication. It is worth repeating that nothing that is being advocated will come into conflict with medical advice and all the suggestions will run happily in parallel with your medication. One exception might be in engaging in the very beneficial outcomes of exercise, when an honest appraisal would put you as more sofa sitter than Olympian. Always a good thing to seek medical advice before starting a new exercise regime.

10

GREAT EXPECTATIONS

My wife, Sally, was brought up in the Christian Brethren. Whilst not the most extreme version of this movement, it could certainly be considered to be a cult, with a dominant, perhaps even domineering, leadership and carefully policed prescriptive rules. As a girl she was not allowed to wash her hair or have friends round on Sundays. In what was probably a significant breach of the rules, her mother took her to see *Mary Poppins* at a nearby cinema. Sally was anxious in case the apocalypse, promised regularly in the teachings of the church, happened whilst watching the film and she was denied a place in heaven.

The church was also extremely misogynistic; women were largely the teamakers, child carers and were required to be silent in the services. In her own family her brothers were encouraged to go to university, whilst the two girls were directed towards the retail sector until they could find a suitable man to take care of them. Fortunately, she broke the mould and had an extremely successful career in nursing. As to whether she found a suitable man to take care of her, I guess I would not be the right person to comment.

Such inappropriate and directive comments will almost certainly have a limiting impact on individuals and beliefs about the future direction of their lives and the options and possibilities.

Comments, both positive and negative, can come from parents, teachers and friends and, almost unconsciously, through presentations on TV and other media as to what success can look like.

BENCHMARK

We are graded and assessed on an almost relentless basis as we go through life. Formal schooling and subsequent education will seek to allocate us into a particular category and trajectory. Peer groups will also lay down markers that define success and provide the boundaries for inclusion and exclusion. For some, these will be corrosively limiting whilst others will approach life with a flamboyance that seeks to impress through such things as opinions, personality and material possessions. However, does it really matter what make of watch you have and, what clothes you wear or what type of car you might drive? For many, such intangible badges of status and positioning can become excessively important. It is not uncommon for people to get into debt as a result of acquisitions made to secure affirmation.

One of the most divisive and damaging periods of education followed World War II. An educationalist, Sir Cyril Burt, who was not only very taken with the idea of IQ but also with eugenics. The latter is about breeding a designer population and ironically this was one of the things that Hitler had been spearheading in Nazi Germany. Burt's work suggested that an educational *sorting hat* could be applied to children at the age of 11 and they could then be allocated to grammar schools or secondary modern schools on the basis of this superficial testing. Families were split as some siblings were deemed to be academic and others in the same family seen to be more vocational. A high percentage of those who attended secondary modern schools left without any qualifications. This was largely because they were understood to lack the capability to excel.

Some years later, researchers re-examined Burt's data and found it to have been falsified. This was even to the extent of Burt making up the names of his co-researchers (Gillie 1977). Many adults have gone through life impoverished by the scars of a period of education and social sorting built on lies.

I worked for several years with educationalist, Dylan Wiliam. At the heart of his thinking lay the idea of formative assessment and feedback. If you think about it, most of the judgements in education come towards the end of the process. At this point our achievements or their lack are a bit like a post mortem, a little late in the day for using the information in order to make future positive changes. We need constructive feedback which we can use to move forward as we understand our strengths and develop.

Wiliam (1999) was dismissive of what he called 'ego feedback'; telling people that they are 'a star', 'you're a hero', 'you are flying', or that you are a 'prince' or 'princess', well the list goes on. Not only are many of these turns of phrase cringeworthy. Such descriptions are largely useless and even damaging as they have no substance or potential for supporting development.

We need to be surrounded by the authentic, people who will say it as it is when we ask or need it. People who have our back and interests centre stage. Ditch the sycophants, avoid the cynics and especially give a wide birth to those whose only interest is self-aggrandisement. The latter will only use you as a step up on their own personal stairway to heaven.

KUBLER ROSS

Elizabeth Kübler-Ross was a Swiss–American psychiatrist and the first individual to transfigure the way that the world looks at the terminally ill. She pioneered hospice care, palliative care, bioethics, and near-death research, and was the first to bring terminally ill individuals' lives to the public eye. Kubler-Ross (1969) put forward the widely accepted five stages of grief, usually described as denial, anger, bargaining, depression and acceptance. Post-2000, this model was been taken on by an increasing number of companies to explain reactions to change and loss.

The following diagram charts the likely process when we deal with planned change, change that we are complicit with. It could be a change in our job, a house move, a new relationship, the birth of a child and even buying a car.

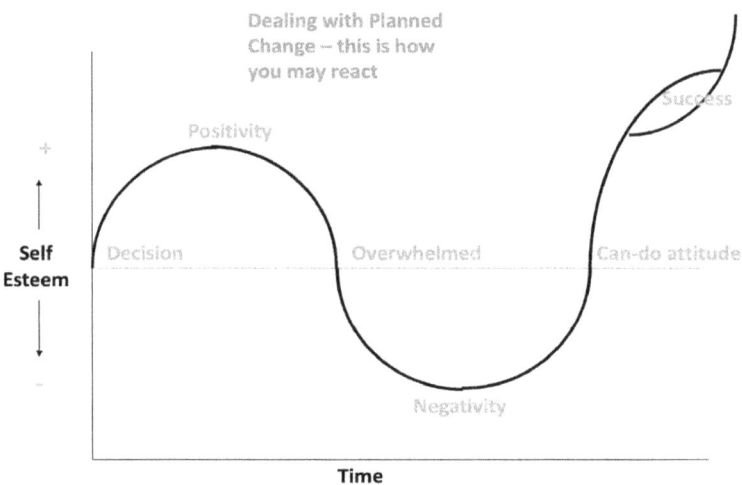

Graph 10.1 *The Emotional change curve (After Kubler-Ross)*

Consider applying for a job, where this particular post represents a step up for you. Following a successful interview you sense considerable positivity and elation. Your self-esteem rises and you tell your friends and others close to you about your success. A short time later, you start to reflect on the consequences of accepting this new post and you begin to engage with the realities of what you have got yourself into. It may be that to take up the post you will have to move, certainly leave establish colleagues behind. You read the job description carefully and there are new skills that you will need to develop.

In this phase of the change curve there is a lot going on and it is common to feel overwhelmed. There is usually a descent into the feelings of negativity, and a reduction in self-esteem. We often get caught by the impostor syndrome. It is a bit like having the pieces of a jigsaw puzzle, but somebody has not given you the box with the picture on top in order to show how it all fits together.

In most cases, over time, we start to make the transition through the stages and formulate a plan as to how we are going to handle these changes. As we do this our self-esteem rises, we develop an increasingly can-do attitude and begin to brace ourselves for the next change. Yes, even the parents of a new-born, who are absolutely delighted with their baby, soon plummet as they begin to wonder what on earth it was they have done. It is normal, it is commonplace, it is the way human beings handle change.

Many have to respond to an imposed change, perhaps a health issue, an unexpected financial situation, or a change in working practice resulting from the restructuring of the organisation that you work for. The change curve still works in this situation though many of the emotions shift. In the initial phase, denial and then anger predominate and perversely the latter can cause us to feel increased self-esteem largely derived from righteous indignation. As this powerful emotion starts to ebb and we have to deal with the complexities of the situation, our bewilderment cuts in and our self-esteem begins to drop. The rise at the other side begins as we accept the situation and cope and even make the best of what we see as difficult circumstances.

When we ride the change curve the hallmarks are really a movement from paralysis to analysis to action.

DEFERRED GRATIFICATION

This refers to the ability to resist immediate rewards or pleasures in order to obtain something more substantive further down the line. It seems to link with self-discipline and impulse control and often requires patience and a clear appreciation of longer-term benefits rather than the instant and often limited rewards. Individuals who practice deferred gratification usually demonstrate better decision-making because of their awareness of the implications of their choices beyond the immediate. People who side step the immediate also tend to be more resilient in the face of the challenges of setbacks as they understand and accept that achieving long-term goals may require some short-term sacrifices.

Developing this trait can be challenging, particularly, in our contemporary society which focuses less on long-term goals and more on the immediate. It involves developing the ability to swim against many of our contemporary currents such as 'buy now' marketing strategies, or some gaming and social media platforms who are heavily connected to the dopamine loop. The capacity for deferred gratification is frequently associated with positive outcomes.

THE CONSTRUCT

Belief is both powerful and extremely difficult to deconstruct. It is cruel to macerate somebody's positive vision of the future.

However sometimes we become confronted with levels of commitment which lack connection with any real form of reality. A friend of mine, who is a GP, was called out to a patient who believed that he had the ability to fly and had tried to do so from his bedroom window. When my friend arrived, he was surprised and relieved to see the patient sitting in an armchair with a cup of tea. All became clear as he realised that the residence was actually a bungalow and the attempts at flight had resulted in nothing more than a sprained ankle. His expectations and beliefs were readjusted.

I ran a training day with some 90 members of the medical profession. The focus was supporting patients locked in a 'can't change, won't change' mindset. Their repeated complaint was that they had given people significant and relevant information and yet still they did not make the necessary changes to improve their health and situation. To make my point I asked these 90 medical professionals if they would participate in a small experiment? With their agreement I use some very simple hypnosis. I asked them to imagine that in the right-hand they were holding the neck of a large balloon, bit by bit this imaginary balloon has been filled with lighter than air helium gas and as that they would feel their arm being lifted by the balloon. The more gas, the more their arm elevated.

Of the 90 participants, approximately 80 ended up sitting with arms in the air. I then reversed the process asking to imagine that the helium was leaking from their balloon and their arm came back down again. This was not a heavy session; people were conscious and aware of what was going on and yet absolutely astonished that an idea could be planted in their heads which would have an observable physical outcome. When we take a construct into our heads the consequences will be far-reaching and will defy rationality.

It is worth reflecting on our self-limiting beliefs and also on beliefs which are ill-founded and which can take us in the wrong direction. Some of these beliefs will permeate our thinking and personality for a lifetime, and some will impair our potential and levels of fulfilment. It is time for some of us to cut the puppet master strings.

As this chapter concludes I have put in a simple daily routine, a sort of flossing for the mind. It is very simple; however, practice it regularly and it will create an uplift of your thinking, attitude and performance.

START AS YOU MEAN TO GO ON – FLOSSING FOR THE MIND

Begin the day with a few moments of gratitude. Could be:-

- family
- a particular friend
- a lovely sunset
- a nice meal the previous evening
- something good about your health

(Actually, there are always lots to choose from)

Perhaps move on to a few affirmations (always first person, present tense and definitely without qualifiers such as: possibly, maybe or perhaps. You do not have to pretend to have super-powers, but this is the time to give mediocrity the elbow. Try a few of these and then go on and create your own:-

- I am having fun today
- I am learning something new
- I am speaking to the person who's been a bit distant

- I am using today to show people what I can do
- I am building on an experience from yesterday
- I am making this a productive day

Finally, ask yourself (just take a minute, two at the most) and answer these questions:-

- Am I really happy?
- If yes, why? If no, why not?
- How could I make myself feel better?
- Is there anything bothering me at the moment?
- What steps will I take to do something about it?

11

HALL OF MIRRORS

Our perception is our reality and is a highly edited version of our engagement with the world we inhabit and the people that we interact with. There is usually a working congruence between our story and other peoples' versions of events. It is this overlap that allows communication and engagement in common enterprises. The way that we structure and tell our stories has a huge impact on the way that we think, conduct relationships and how we make decisions. Put people together and the stories and anecdotes start to roll. We are hard wired to tell stories. Just stand in the queue in the building society or post office and listen. Relatively few customers limit themselves to their simple transaction. Many embellish their fiscal exchange with stories about their journey, the weather, grandchildren and even their health (or more usually its lack). Post–toddling children delight in transfixing consenting adults with accounts of their exploits. This could all become very philosophical and take us down a serious rabbit-hole labelled truth. As Napoleon Bonaparte allegedly said *'History is the version of past events that people have decided to agree upon'* (French general & politician 1769-1821), but then he said a lot of things.

So why are stories so much a part of our human existence? There are probably two major drivers; firstly, our need for significance and context and secondly, the need to order or make sense of our private world.

DO YOU KNOW WHO I AM?

Usually when people meet, they try to find connection with each other. Consider for a moment going to a party. As strangers meet, questions begin to flow; "How do you know Anne and Mike?" "What do you do for a living?" "Do you live locally?" and "Do you have a family?". If connection is made through these questions and the subsequent storytelling, then the embryonic relationship continues. If the links are not made, then the individuals tend to move on to other victims of their relentless enquiry. We like people who are like us or people who are like who we would like to be like. Denning (2007) argued that 'dogs sniff each other and humans tell stories!' Personally, I am happy that it is that way round. Denning also noted:

> Physical science has had an aversion to anything to do with storytelling in part because it deals with such murky things as intentions, emotions and matters of the heart. Yet in the past couple of decades, most of the human sciences have grasped the centrality of narrative to human affairs. Narrative has come to be influential in vast regions of psychology, anthropology, philosophy, sociology, political theory, literary studies, religious studies, psychotherapy and even medicine. Management is amongst the last of the disciplines to recognise the central significance of narrative to the issues that it deals with. (2011, p. 11)

There is a belief that we are connected, if not directly then at the distance of a few interpersonal steps. This idea came from the work of psychologist Stanley Milgram (1967). He randomly selected the names of 160 people living in Omaha, Nebraska and sent each one a packet with the name and address of a stockbroker who worked in Boston and lived in Sharon, Massachusetts. They were asked to put their own name on the packet and then mail it to someone they knew who was closer geographically. When the packet arrived Milgram noted how many people had been involved in the chain. Typically, most packets involved a chain of some five or six individuals to get the packet to its destination. It is from this experiment that we get the idea of six degrees of separation and lends some substance to the view that it is indeed a small world.

Stories and their truncated relatives, anecdotes are the vehicles for establishing connection. Paradoxically excessively complex, disconnected or long drawn-out stories actually break connections between people.

MY PERCEPTION IS MY REALITY

The second driver of our need to tell stories relates to how we order our private world. We frequently define this by telling stories. Some people struggle with the idea of their experience being considered in these terms. They believe that their account of the world is stable, objective and corresponds with the experience of others. In fact, nothing could be further from the truth.

The story we live in has an extremely significant impact on the way in which we think. Our ordering of our experience changes the way in which we perform, how we process challenge, how we make decisions, the information that we collect and even our physiology at the cellular level throughout our bodies. Pert (1997) commented:

'It's well documented, for example, that people have more heart attacks on Monday mornings (when the work week begins) than any other day of the week, and that death rates peak during the days after Christmas for Christians and after Chinese New Year for the Chinese. Since these are all days with high emotional valence, one way or another, it seems clear that the emotions in some way correlate with the state of people's hearts' (p. 189).

Our mental state and the narrative that we engage with significantly affects our performance. Two Dutch researchers Dijksterhuis and van Knippenberg (1998) asked a group of students to answer forty-two questions taken from the game 'Trivial Pursuit'. Before answering the questions half were asked to think about soccer hooligans and the other half about university professors. They were allotted five minutes and asked to write down what came to mind. Immediately after they answered the test questions, the former scoring 42.6% and the latter 55.6%.

Steele and Aronson (1995) conducted research with American African Caribbean college students. The test was taken from the Graduate Record Examination and was preceded with a simple pre-test, which collected some basic personal data and which also included some details on ethnic background. The mere engagement with these basic questions evoked negative stereotypes, which cut the test scores by half.

These research-based examples graphically illustrate the reduction in performance when negative frames of reference or story impact our thinking, Consider how our own performance might deteriorate if we are repeatedly exposed to negative messages about ourselves, or if such a message is given to us by someone we trust. We should not expect to be cosseted and insulated from challenge, but there is a need to explore ways that messages and feedback are communicated constructively and certainly not carelessly. There are so many examples where corrosive feedback has damaged people, damaging their performance and even leading to breakdown or disengagement.

Our adoption of negative stories changes our thinking at a profound level. Our brains are wonderfully sophisticated, but their core processes are linked to securing our survival. Imagine for a moment that you are sat on the beach on a warm afternoon; you can hear the sound of the sea and your hand is clutching a glass of chilled Pinot Grigio. If that is an attractive scenario, then you would need little encouragement to linger in that situation. If you are confronted by a negative perception of yourself, for example working for a coercive employer with the empathy and compassion of a house-brick you will feel uncomfortable and find some way out of the situation. However, many of us become fearful and this gets overridden by professional pride, a feeling that things might turn a corner or an array of financial pressures you stand your ground. The survival mechanisms rooted in your brain will now turn up the volume and sharpen the contrast. Literally, what was bad becomes portrayed as even worse in an attempt to get you to take action.

One of the key changes that begins to emerge from this state is 'all or nothing thinking'. 'When you are stressed, your brain works differently. You are more likely to resort to 'All or Nothing' thinking, which causes catastrophising and narrows your focus which makes solving complex problems even more difficult.. In turn this causes more arousal, or stress and so continues the 'loop' exhausting you' (Elliott and Tyrrell, 2003. p. 18)

One fascinating example of how our chain-linking of fragments of our story can change our whole perspective is catastrophisation. My all-time favourite illustration must be this homely domestic interchange between my wife, Sally and myself. However, once you are aware of how it operates you will notice that it is commonplace in the stories that we hear and indeed those that we tell ourselves.

Our eldest son, then in his mid-twenties, had been made redundant. He had been applying for jobs and on this particular day had a promising interview with a local firm. I had been working in London and arrived back home around 10.30pm desperate for a sit down and something to eat. The dialogue went like this:

(Me) 'How did David get on? Did he get the job?'

(Sally) 'No, it was a real shame, he didn't get the job. Of course, these are difficult times with the economy. Nobody's got jobs. David will never get a job. He'll never leave home and you won't be able to retire and you'll die.'

This was spectacular especially as the whole conversation was on the doorstep and took less than 40 seconds. This was catastrophising at its best (or worst?). Even though our narratives may not be real – and even current – they have the capacity to amplify and generate stress. Our thinking is not objective and needs to be managed.

In fact, most situations that we experience are probably not particularly extreme. There are elements of good and bad in them. A recent holiday in Cyprus was good if you discounted the three days of torrential rain and the fourteen-hour thunderstorm in the middle. If you lose this broader and more balanced picture circumstances are viewed through distorting lenses and even your language changes, Elliott and Tyrrell (2003) have identified the following key words that indicate if someone is engaging in this kind of thinking: -

Always	Never	Perfect
Impossible	Awful	Terrible
Ruined	Disastrous	Furious

Table 11.1 Words that Indicate 'All or Nothing Thinking' (p. 45)

When we allow our thinking to become distorted in this way situations can rapidly invoke despair. The difficult colleague becomes a 'psychopath' or 'impossible', an overdraft is restated as 'bankruptcy', the car battery going flat signals the collapse of the car's complete electrical system. The list goes on and on. This is not to trivialise the difficult situations that we can and probably will face in life. We must have mechanisms to check out our distorting perception.

Some years ago I was told the story of a lady who lived near a park, though I cannot remember who told it to me. She routinely exercised her dog there each morning. As often happens with regular dog walkers she soon became on nodding terms with a number of other regulars. There was one exception, an older lady who never responded to her greeting. In fact, she completely ignored any comment. This went on for several years and each day the greeting was rebuffed, despite being delivered with greater volume and intensity. Our dog walker was about to move from the area and decided to have one last attempt at getting a response. Still nothing. In desperation, she confronted the older lady and asked her why, over several years, she had been so rude? The older lady looked very embarrassed and apologised profusely explaining that her eyesight was not particularly good and that her hearing was even worse. A misunderstanding with a valid explanation had been transformed into something quite different. The older lady had been vilified and our dog walker carried an increasing burden of resentment. A story badly constructed which had come to be believed as inviolate truth.

Back in 2002 the influential educational writer and good friend, John West-Burnham had talked about leaders needing to have an 'internal personal reservoir of hope'. His words have a much wider application beyond leadership. This was described as having a calm centre at the heart of the individual from which their values and vision flow and which continues to enable effective interpersonal engagement and sustainability of personal self–belief in the face of not only day to day pressures but critical incidents. I would argue that at the core of the concept of hope is an underpinning positive story, which provides a 'reservoir' both for us as individuals, but which is a buoyancy aid for those around us. Conversely, when we hold on to a negative story this could be equated with the ebbing of hope. It will result in the change in our thought patterns along the lines that have been described. Our negativity will be recognised by others and our personal circle will diminish.

THE GOOD BOOK

Many of us receive all too few positive comments. It sometimes seems that some of the people around us have 'grown out' of the ability to praise. None of us will benefit from plastic praise or the acclaim of sycophants but like all human beings we do thrive on positive feedback. If we occupy a position of responsibility, then it is probable that like the carving at the top of the totem pole we will be in receipt of more bird droppings than those further down. It can certainly feel that way as we try to work with people to a good purpose.

A practical strategy is to keep a 'Good Book'. This is a simple personal scrapbook. In this you place those letters of thanks, record those positive comments and incidents from other people. Turning its pages on dark cheerless days that inevitably come in life will help restore perspective. Banal? Perhaps it is, but then not everything good has to be sophisticated.

The first of two favourites is from my youngest son:

Dad you are one of my favourite parents.

The other, more serious is from an ex-student that I supervised, probably the most moving comment that I have ever received:

Though the journey has been tough, he's put good people along the way to help me. I am happy and very fortunate that our paths should cross. My parents saved my life; you saved my soul. I learnt a lot from you, not just about leadership but about myself and about the meaning of life. You have spotted my weaknesses which you politely never brought up. Instead, you've always been encouraging and built my confidence, which I lost many years ago. You've led me to value myself. When I return home there may be a tough road ahead of me. But I believe in myself and remain positive, I will get through it all.

I hope that that was not too personal, but it does it for me.

HOLDING YOUR OWN

Most people like to think that they are fair and open-minded, ready to be convinced by another person's point of view. This is a commendable position but one, which is sadly at odds with our day to day, experience. People seem to be able to hold on to viewpoints with incredible tenacity in the face of contradictory information and leaders are no different. Many of us have known for a long time that other people do this; perhaps it is the moment to reflect on our personal aptitude for bias. It may well be that our beliefs and opinions are closely wedded to who we are as people.

Consider two people arguing as to whether they would rather drive a Volkswagen or a Kia. Certainly, technical information might come into the discussion: performance, customer satisfaction surveys, fuel economy and acceleration etc. The reality is that they are both good cars and yet a comment such as 'I wouldn't be seen dead in' (insert the vehicle of choice here) is not an impressive indicator of our cognitive processing. The science fiction writer, Robert Heinlein (1953), noted, 'Man is not a rational animal, he is a rationalizing animal' (p.27).

More recently this ability of human beings to defend their particular position or own brand of thinking has been explored by psychologists. Lord, Ross and Lepper (1979) presented subjects with evidence supporting or rejecting the effectiveness of capital punishment to a mixed group of subjects holding divergent views on the subject. In fact, they selected twenty-four protagonists and the same number of antagonists. The research team hypothesized that each opposing group would use the same pieces of evidence to further support their opinions. After reading the article on capital punishment the subjects were given detailed research descriptions of the study they had just read, but this time it included procedures, results and prominent criticisms shown in a table or graph. They were then asked to evaluate the study, stating how well it was conducted and how convincing they found the evidence.

The results were in line with the researchers' hypothesis; in fact, there was even greater polarization of views amongst some participants than had been expected. Students found that studies, which supported their pre-existing view were superior to those which contradicted it, in a number of detailed and specific ways. In fact, the studies all described the same experimental procedure but with only the purported result changed. Overall, there was a visible increase in the polarization of opinion. Initial analysis of the experiment shows that proponents and opponents confessed to shifting their attitudes slightly in the direction of the first study they read. Once subjects read the more detailed study, they returned to their original belief regardless of the evidence provided, pointing to the details that supported their viewpoint and disregarding anything that was to the contrary. This is termed confirmation bias.

Even more intriguing was the study undertaken by Westen et al (2006). Functional neuroimaging (fMRI) was used to study a sample of committed Democrats and Republicans during the three months prior to the U.S. Presidential Elections of 2004. Each group was given the task of considering threatening or contradictory information relating to their candidate of choice; John Kerry or George Bush respectively. During the task the subjects were scanned to see what parts of their brain were active.

The fMRI showed emotional areas of the brain activated but did not see any increased activation of the parts of the brain normally engaged during reasoning. Instead, they saw a network of emotion-based circuits lighting up, including circuits hypothesized to be involved in regulating emotion, and areas linked to resolving conflicts.

Participants returned to their biased conclusions and found ways to discard rational information to sustain their own position. Of course, the discrediting information related to the opposing candidate was gratefully received. Once their preferred bias had been restored the brain rewarded itself with a secretion of dopamine. This would produce a pleasant high and would therefore confirm the 'rightness' of moving back to their original and preferred position.

It is fascinating watching a rerun of this with the growing indictment of Donald Trump. The charges seem to escalate and be matched in turn by the increasing support of his adherents.

The inclusion of this research into confirmation bias is not about engendering self–doubt or undermining self–confidence. It is about arguing that we should all ensure that systems are in place to check our views, policies, vision and perceptions. In Alice's Adventures in Wonderland (Carroll, 2014) Alice reflects on her changing experiences and comments:

> I know who I WAS when I got up this morning, but I think I must have been changed several times since then.

Controlling our personal narrative by reframing or not rushing to complete the story is a powerful support to our wellbeing. Our perceptions of events and even ourselves are often distorted by the comments of others, the story that we are living in and particularly by stress, especially if it is sustained. Perhaps there are good reasons to see our images of ourselves and our interpretations of events as being like a trip through a fairground's distorting hall of mirrors or if you are GenZ using apps like ToonMe to change pictures. However, just because you can put a beard on your Granny, it does not mean it is real, assuming, of course, that she has not actually got one.

Humans have, as far as we can tell, a unique ability to ruminate about the past and project possible scenarios into the future. Even though these may not be real – and certainly they will not be current – they have the capacity to reset our emotions, especially if they are negative. PTSD provides a powerful example of how time-distanced events can drive the now. Catastrophisation needs to be eliminated. If you find yourself going down this line, pause and then commit to coming up with at least three alternative scenarios that you could use to describe the situation. Ambiguity can be of great benefit in dialling down inappropriate certainties that we may have and hold. The more that we can say 'maybe', the greater will be the range of resources that are likely to be available to us; this is in contrast with concrete certainty, which narrows our focus and will marshal a particular set of resources to effect a specific course of action. This runs counter to the narrowing impact of stress, which tries to move us towards 'all- or-nothing thinking'.

This Chinese fable makes this point and also demonstrates how stories can engage with us emotionally as well:

> Once there was a farmer who had a handsome and strong horse. The horse was not only beautiful to look at but helped supply the income on which the man and his family depended.
>
> But one night, the horse escaped and ran off. All the other villagers were deeply sympathetic towards the farmer and his loss. They came to offer their condolences at such a massive loss.

'What a terrible thing to have happened,' they said to the man. But he just shrugged and calmly said, 'Maybe...or maybe not.' They were surprised at his attitude, sangfroid and nonchalance, and soon went about their day.

A few days later, the farmer's beautiful stallion returned with 12 beautiful mares in tow. This was a real bonus.

All the locals were quick to congratulate him. 'What wonderful luck for you!' they cried. But again, the man, chilled to the core, said: 'Well... maybe...or maybe not. Let's wait and see, shall we?' Once more, the villagers were nonplussed by his attitude but felt pleased for him anyway.

The very next day, the man's son was taming one of the wild horses when he fell and broke his leg. 'What bad luck!' cried the villagers. 'Maybe it's good luck; maybe it's bad luck. We'll have to wait and see.' said the man.

'Really?' said the villagers, who were getting tired of his apparent fatalism. 'Please tell us, how on earth can your son breaking his leg not be considered to be bad luck!?' And they went about their business.

But just a few days later, royal messengers came to the village proclaiming that all young men were to be immediately drafted into the army for the purpose of serving in an unjust and, as it turned out, hopeless and destructive war. But the man's son, having just broken his leg, was rejected for service. The entire company he would have enlisted with soon perished in one of the very first assaults of the war.

All the other villagers came to the old man and now said, 'Whew, what good luck that your son was spared fighting and being killed in the war!' The man just smiled, but they knew what he was thinking.

(Author Unknown)

The farmer in the fable is depicted as someone who does not assume – or, more importantly, does not catastrophise – but waits to see the emerging truth of the situation. Uncertainty is not the same as ambiguity. The former is about indecision, the latter is about not rushing to fill the meaning vacuum. I would suggest, as an aside, that if we have children, 'ambiguity' is one of the greatest gifts that we can give them.

12

STRATEGIC SELFISHNESS

Family friends, Roger and Jo, went to work for a year in Canada. At the time their children were quite young, a toddler and a pram-bound younger child. Jo, a stranger in a strange town, took the children for a walk to the nearby shops. Her family outing was suddenly interrupted by the screech of tyres from a fast-moving car. Looking round, she saw the vehicle travelling at speed towards her, with the driver losing control. In fact, these were armed robbers being chased by a marked police car. She hurled herself forward and pushed the toddler and the pram out of the path of the speeding getaway car. The children were safe, but she sustained horrific injuries especially to the head and face. She survived but the scars of the incident remained evident many years later.

Just maybe, the cynical might dismiss this as an instinctive maternal act. Personally, I have always thought that this was inspirational story which ranks amongst the many that demonstrate self-sacrifice and altruism. Such acts offer a counterbalance to atrocities and the wanton disregard with which our planet home can be treated.

The fusion writer, Ricard, (2015) offers a compelling argument for altruism. Coming from a Buddhism perspective alongside a deep engagement with psychology he suggests:

In the contemporary world, though, altruism is more than ever a necessity, even an urgent one. It is also a natural manifestation of human kindness for which we all have potential, despite multiple, often selfish, motivations that run through and sometimes dominate our minds. (2015, p. 10)

If we did a 'hands up' for who would like to be treated with greater kindness, then I would be a frontrunner. However, is it that simple, do we just need to populate the world with nicer people? Dickens (1843) in his novella *A Christmas Carol* presents us with the self-consumed Ebeneezer Scrooge. Despite the ultimate acts of redemption, it presents an ugly portrait of unbridled selfishness. Board a long-haul flight and a more balanced message is broadcast. In that safety presentation, there is always the instruction that in the event of the depressurisation of the cabin you should put the dangling oxygen mask on yourself first. Then you are free to help others. Anoxia is not a great platform from which to support others.

HARDENING OF THE OUGHTERIES

The suggestion here is that it is not about a choice between self-sacrifice and selfishness, but is more about the management of our resources. Of course, there will be times when we run on the red line of our personal limits. A sleep deprived parent does not ration attention to a crying baby. I did not leave my own father's bedside when he was dying. Perhaps, a more prosaic example is flooring the mental accelerator whilst revising for an exam. However, it is common for many people to give of themselves beyond their operating limits. Sustained mental and physical overload will almost inevitably have consequences such as stress, anxiety and even auto immune diseases to name but a few.

It is worth reflecting regularly on the drivers that are pushing us into untenable lifestyles. Frequently, we are being propelled by the demands of others. Some of these may be overt, such as a callous and unthinking line manager or an overbearing and excessively demanding parent. There are also ingrained thought patterns perhaps from our parents, school or a values explicit organisation such as a church. These internalised thought patterns will often surface in our internal dialogue as 'ought' or 'should'. They seem to engage with an external and sometimes non-specific reference point that draws us into a belief that a particular course of action should be self–evident. If we can add a mixer of guilt into the cocktail, then a really toxic thought pattern can ensue.

In straightforward terms, impositions by others can confer victim status on us. As soon as others are defining us and our behaviour, or we lose our ability to make our own choices, we are surrendering control to others. The pressure may start to build as we feel resentment about such control or, if we are compliant, then we will have sacrificed our identity in some way.

The Canadian psychiatrist, Eric Berne (1978), was fascinated by human interactions. He developed insights into how these operated, developing his theories as 'Transactional Analysis' (TA). The core was that each of us has within us archetypes, a battery of stored resources that we can draw on when we interact socially. One was deemed 'adult', where we are working with others in a state of rational, respectful mutuality. He also invoked the categories of 'adapted child' and 'adapted parent'. The former can involve playfulness and creativity but can also cause us to adopt a dependent stance where we want others to solve our problems. The archetype known as the 'adapted parent' is when we draw on the style of significant others such as parents and teachers. We move to stamp our authority on others and take control.

A fascinating spin-off from Berne's work, and one which provides a useful perspective in understanding the games that people play with us, is Karpman's work (1972). It is usually titled as The Karpman Triangle or more frequently as The Drama Triangle. Forrest (2008) provides the following summary:

> The three roles on the victim triangle are Persecutor, Rescuer and Victim. Karpman placed these three roles on an inverted triangle and described them as being the three aspects or faces of victim. No matter where we may start out on the triangle, victim is where we end up; therefore no matter what role we are in on the triangle, we are in victimhood. If we are on the triangle we're living as victims, plain and simple! (2008, p. 1)

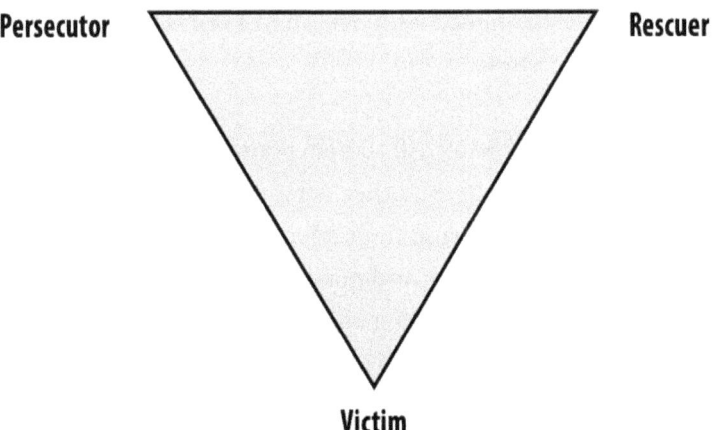

Fig. 12.1 The Drama (or Karpman) Triangle

The model suggests that in many interpersonal transactions people tend to adopt one of these basic positions. Forrest holds that most people have a primary style. She describes this as a 'starting gate', rather like describing our handedness. So, for example, a 'starting gate rescuer' will tend to identify with this role in engaging with another person. However, once on the triangle, the individuals will rotate through the all of the positions, going completely around the triangle, sometimes in a matter of minutes, or even seconds, many times every day.

Victim. This is a position of helplessness and the appeal that they make to others is to request their assistance. This approach to relationships probably has its roots in the person's childhood where such behaviours were used as a means to gain attention. The Victim, if not actually being persecuted, will often seek out a 'persecutor' and also a 'rescuer', that person who will save the day but also perpetuate their victimhood. It has a great deal of resonance with Seligman's (1972) research into Learned Helplessness.

Rescuer. There will be a rush to help people and situations but they can often confirm the other person in a state of dependency. Crucially, by focusing their energy on someone else they can avoid their own issues and personal anxiety. Their actions are all too often disguised as a concern for the victim's needs.

Persecutor. Their response is to project blame and criticism into the situation, often coupled with aggression. There is a strong element of control and authority linked with the position. Perhaps as result of being abused in earlier life, there is a tendency to make a pre-emptive strike.

It is a little like the board game played in the 1995 film *Jumanji*. The film centres on a board game which rapidly changes from pastime to panic. One of the characters, Alan Parrish, becomes trapped in the game itself. 26 years later in 1995, siblings Judy and Peter Shepherd find the game, begin playing and then unwittingly release the now-adult Alan. The gang resolve to finish the game in order to reverse all the destruction it has caused.

If someone engages in a dialogue from one of the positions, they are inviting us to join their game. If we accept, we can only take up one of the unused positions and, just as in the fictitious board game *Jumanji*, we are now trapped in making a series of potentially endless moves. For example, if the other person takes up the 'victim' position we can enter the dialogue as either a 'rescuer' or as a 'persecutor'. The problem begins to emerge when the 'victim' feels unhappy with their role and changes position. If we have been drawn in as the 'rescuer' the only space available to them is that of the 'persecutor' and suddenly our helping response feels as if it is being thrown back in our faces. The positions now begin to rotate round the triangle like some distressing pavane.

The Drama Triangle provides an analysis of behaviours. Of course, we are not immune from initiating interactions in this way ourselves. However, we are unlikely to get out of this unproductive and often fraught way of conducting relationships unless we know that we are on the triangle. As we become more aware of our own tendencies, we can train ourselves not to join the game when we enter dialogue with others and turn off this distracting and draining approach to communications. We will also recognise when we are being baited to join the game by others and decline to engage. A person, even a friend, who demands action and hints at a problem which you have either created or at one which they think you should have solved can be disarmed with a question as to their responsibility or suggestion or even by a deferred response. They may well move to another position, perhaps that of persecutor, and then spin impotently round the positions. You, meanwhile, have not entered into any 'spur of the moment' commitment to solve the issue and have not been drawn into an unstable discourse.

This model is extremely useful in understanding how people can interreact and how apparently straightforward situations can sour. If our tendency is to try and sort out other people and their problems. If we cover for others, pay their bills, bail them out of trouble over and over, do their work for them, we are taking responsibility for them. When we take care of others at our own expense and that means the victim role will be our next stop. This quite different from being responsible to others. The difference is simple yet profound. Being responsible to others is something that happens as a natural consequence of taking responsibility for ourselves. Whereas, when we take responsibility for others, we can easily neglect ourselves.

Back to the triangle, in full flow we can end up in any of the three positions. If we are a 'starting gate rescuer' then we are increasing the risk of becoming overwhelmed. As the game moves further, the 'rescuer' frequently finds their interventions spark tension and hostility.

JUST SAY NO

It is so often easier to say yes. The conversation will almost certainly be more pleasant, we will experience, if only briefly, the feeling of being wanted, or perhaps even being valued. The subsequent reflection can be a little like being the victim of time share sale, what seemed to be a good idea at the time has now become a source of anxiety.

Make a list of ten people who you see on a regular basis; perhaps best to consider those where the contact is voluntary. Consider which ones routinely leave you feeling irritated or even demeaned. What would happen if you simply said no to the next invitation to meet up? When someone wants to borrow your hedge trimmer and returned it last time with the cable severed, why would you lend it again?

When we use the word 'no' we are recognising that we understand our limits. This is not about refusing to help a friend with a real need but about evaluating our own resources. The closer and more frequently we get to setting and maintaining these the stronger and less stressed we become.

Of course, the word 'no' does register more powerfully than its antonym 'yes'. Using the word 'no' can have a cost but surprisingly often that cost is a lot less than a compliant and ill considered 'yes'. This is not about creating a mandate to be rude. A negative response can be carefully and even sensitively packaged. Drawing on the previous section, if you are a 'starting gate rescuer' a positive response is potentially a significant threat to your wellbeing.

STRATEGIC SELFISHNESS

Some people will have found this chapter quite challenging to read, they have based many of their relationships on being a person who is there for others. The thought of making changes brings with it a fear of possible rejection. Whilst this is understandable, strategic selfishness is not the polar opposite of being altruistic. Rather, it means that we make careful choices about how we deploy our (limited) resources. We decide when to expend them and when they should be conserved.

It is by taking an overview of how we interact with people and situations that our decisions are not fogged by the anoxia of the demands of others.

Has compassion been eroded? In no way; in fact our responses to others become more considered, more targeted and more appropriate. We have not allowed our engagement with other people to be diluted by being overstretched.

Forrest offers this observation:

> I believe that every dysfunctional interaction, in relationship with other or self, takes place on the victim triangle. But until we become conscious of these dynamics, we cannot transform them. And unless we transform them, we cannot move forward on our journey towards re-claiming emotional, mental and spiritual well-being. (2008, p. 1)

13

THE BLIND WOODTURNER

I still enjoy playing some of those early Straits songs, and I'm proud of what we did, and certainly we had some great times. It's what we all wanted when we were kids. But you've got to have the resilience to ride that thing, to pick up that ball and run with it. Because you will keep picking it up and keep running.

(Mark Knopfler)

I was reading a magazine and came across a profile article about Chris Fisher, The Blind Woodturner. There was so much in that title that simultaneously intrigued and terrified me. So, a bit of context here. Woodturning involves spinning a piece of wood, often a square section and shaping it into aesthetically pleasing products by using a sharp pointy steel tool.

At the time I was recording a podcast (2022) and asked him for an interview. Chris went totally blind over a couple of weeks as a result toxoplasmosis. Devastating; before going blind he worked as an engineer, rode a motorbike and was learning to fly. However, Chris has always been a big fan of Halloween and wanted a wooden stake for his Dracula tableau. As you do. So, he turned a stake and began woodturning. Several years on and he exhibits his work in a gallery and it is up there with the best, with almost a ceramic-like appearance. Always one to move on to the next level he teaches woodturning, his first student having some movement limitations as a result of cerebral palsy.

Just maybe, I have jumped forward a tad. After losing his sight Chris had to adapt to living in a new way. There were also a number of years of debilitating anxiety. In the early days of turning, he told me that he spent quite a lot of time looking for pieces that had flown off his lathe. The reality was an extremely challenging journey. He pays testimony to the support of family and friends and particularly his wife Nicola. Hope for Chris has been mined with effort and sustained resilience.

As a child, (OK, I will come clean, I was an adult), I liked watching the Roadrunner cartoons. They usually featured dire reprisals by Roadrunner, a fast-running flightless bird, against the predator, Wile E Coyote. At the more sadistic end of the spectrum, the latter was driven into the ground with a hammer, rather like a fence post.

There is currently a great deal of interest in resilience and indeed in running courses to build it with employees and children in schools. However, much of the input is generated by the workplace that is sponsoring the course. All sorts of organisations appear to drive individuals into the ground, like Roadrunner pounding Coyote. Frequently, this resilience 'training' can become the equivalent of providing Coyote with a steel helmet so that the assault can carry on for longer. The outcome of a lot of this training appears to be an attempt to keep people going for longer, whilst not turning reformatting their context. It would seem that training and other initiatives focused on resilience often seek to kick the can down the road in terms of the consequences of working in overheated workplaces and teams. Even in families, if you keep doing what you always did you will get what you always got.

DEFINING RESILIENCE

Literature and films are often based around an individual's struggle against the odds. The 2015 film, *The Revenant*, is very much of that genre. It is about the resilience and fortitude of the hero, Glass, who faces a Native American attack, shelters from the elements in an eviscerated horse carcass, and endures self- surgery and near-suffocation.

It is suggested that a useful working definition of resilience might be: 'the capacity to resist being stalled by adversity'. The following is a more elaborated definition, which can serve as a platform for developing personal resilience:

> Resilience is the ability to modulate and constructively harness the stress response – a capacity essential to both physical and mental health.
>
> Success can hinge on resilience. Setbacks are part of any endeavour and those who act productively will make the most progress.
>
> A person can boost his or her resilience. Strategies include reinterpreting negative events, enhancing positive emotions, becoming physically fit, accepting challenges, maintaining a close social network and imitating resilient role models. (Southwick and Charney, 2013, p. 34)

FOUR CORNERSTONES OF RESILIENCE

When it comes to resilience, we are unlikely to start from a common position. Some of us will have a proven track record of being resilient whilst others amongst us are, perhaps, more vulnerable to being derailed when negative events collude against us. There is no absolute 'index of resilience' and how we respond to adversity can also vary with our personal circumstances, our health, tiredness and age. There is no gold standard but all of us can change the odds in favour of increasing our personal resilience. Again, returning to the core theme of this book of stress reduction across extended periods of time, this also holds true for resilience. However, focusing more specifically on resilience, there are four areas which would benefit from our reflection and development:

Reframing: This connects with Chapter 11– 'Hall of Mirrors' . The point has been made that we make sense of our experience by casting or framing it as a story. If we allow this, subtly or even precipitously, to move to a negative or even catastrophic narrative then our ability to cope within a situation will be damaged. Oschner *et al* (2004) found that the review of a negatively perceived event, so that it is seen in less negative terms tends to change our positive physiological and psychological reactions. Imagine going for a job interview and not getting the much-hoped-for post. Our common reaction is to defend ourselves by constructing a negative account of what happened, and perhaps become hostile to the selection process and to those involved in it. However, taking time to reflect and change the narrative to a more constructive account will reduce our stress. None of us likes to feel rejected and we will rapidly build a story around situations which generate such feelings: 'They didn't give me the chance to explain my strengths'; 'It was a foregone conclusion, they already had somebody else lined up'; 'If only I hadn't stumbled when I answered that one question'; and perhaps most damaging of all, 'Of course, I am not good enough to gain this type of job'.

What would a reframe look like? You could look at the

interview as a learning process. It might be helpful to consider if there were any areas of your skills or experience that the interview has highlighted and which would benefit from development. Reflect on any interactions that you had with other candidates – were there tips or ideas that you could use? Suddenly your defensive posture goes, a positive frame is established, and you will feel your energy and resolve returning. These are key components of resilience; you will begin to recharge.

This is reframing. It leads to an increase in wellbeing and steers you away from bitterness and cynicism, both of which are emotional vampires. Feder *et al* (2008) interviewed 30 former Vietnam prisoners of war about how they now viewed their wartime experiences. Many had reframed their imprisonment, which, for some, had included ill treatment and torture. These ex-prisoners of war had found ways of understanding it such that they had become wiser, stronger and even more resilient. They also recorded that they were better able to see possibilities for the future, relate to others and appreciate life.

> Resilience is associated with realistic optimism, not the rose-coloured form. Because the latter often involves ignoring negative information, people who adopt an overly buoyant outlook tend to underestimate stressful and risky situations. On the other hand, realistic optimists filter out unnecessary negative information but pay close attention to bad news that is relevant to dealing with adversity. (Southwick and Charney, 2013, pp. 38-39)

This is not always an easy to do, but reducing stress will help considerably. Moving from a single strongly held story to exploring a range of possibilities will reduce the possibility of you becoming trapped in the narrative. The option of being locked in a bitter cycle of self-denigratory account of events is a dark and distorting venue. Realistic Optimism could lead us to the point where we decide to withdraw from a particular situation. However, excessive and unanchored optimism is likely to leave our ashes in the smouldering ruin of a given situation.

Social network: A particularly effective way to increase our individual resilience is to maintain a wide-ranging and supportive social network. Please note that these are not virtual friendships! Having a high level of social support has been associated with better psychological outcomes from many types of trauma, including childhood sexual abuse and even the horrors of warfare. In a 1998 study by King et al it was found that returning war veterans who maintained a good social network had significantly lower levels of stress and suffered less from post-traumatic stress disorder than did isolates.

The same findings have been found in a wide range of disparate social groupings, including college students, new mothers, parents of children with serious illnesses, widows and unemployed workers. Knowing that you are backed by others is powerful because it supports self-esteem and personal confidence and is a lifeline if we slip. People with a secure social network demonstrate higher levels of self-belief and, as a consequence, will be more likely to engage actively in problem-solving.

Emotional turbulence: Significant life events are inevitable, though some people appear to believe that their emotions are Teflon-coated and that they will not be impacted by these. The list of these events is considerable: death of a parent, the birth of a child, divorce, ill health, moving to a new house or flat, changing your job, a child leaving home, change in your financial status, getting a speeding ticket, or changing your job. It is important to reflect on the potential impact of these and not underestimate the effect that they can have. My own mother was 85 when she died; I was 55 and married with three children and working as an education consultant. As a family, we enjoyed good relationships with my mother, who lived nearby. She had a relatively short but serious illness before her death. I rationalised her death as timely. Well, you can fill in the clichés. With the value of hindsight I believe that I seriously underestimated the impact of such a significant life event.

When facing bereavement – or indeed, in any of the other situations that I have listed – your resilience will be recalibrated. If we suspect that this is happening, it can be helpful to work with a good coach or an appropriate counsellor. Certainly, *'Time is a great healer'*, but an awful lot can happen while you are waiting.

Good role models: A Canadian psychologist, Bandura (1963), advocated a social learning theory, where he argued that new behaviours can be acquired by observing and imitating others. He stated that learning takes place in a social context, and, further, that it can take place purely through observation without direct instruction.

If we apply Bandura's theory to developing our own resilience, then we need to identify people who model resilience. Because there is a downtime with resilience – that is, there are periods in people's lives when resilience is not being called for – it is suggested that you select about six people for your watching brief. It is likely that someone out of the six will be passing through the sort of context where resilience will be required. It is not clandestine; it does not require camouflage and binoculars. It is useful to develop an authentic relationship with these people and develop this relationship to the point where you can not only observe without stalking them but be able to discuss their situation and their responses without embarrassment.

If you set your strategy for developing your own resilience within the wider context of stress reduction, then by using the techniques explained throughout this book you will be surprised at how resilience develops. This is not a nicety, but rather it is the right platform from which to advance both your personal and professional lives.

BENEFIT FRAUD

The concept of resilience is hard to define and yet it is increasingly understood as being important. It appears that resilience is a multi-facete.d and unstable construct. Perhaps it is fragility of people following the pandemic that is highlighting the desirability of resilience as a trait. Like many aspects of human personality this is likely to be a synthesis of nature and nurture; the weighting of cause underlying resilience is difficult to establish. For many of us, workload and the unreasonable expectations that we believe are being imposed on us impacts our personal sustainability. Many of our children have emergent problems with resilience. Perhaps this is because many are excessively protected in early childhood and then move rapidly to inhabit a digital world where failure and disaster can be resolved by a reset.

Human beings are not designed to perform at the outer reaches of endurance on a continual basis. They need ups and downs, excitement and rest. Driving themselves – or being driven by others – to work flat out all the time leads to breakdown and collapse. Today's uncivilized workplace culture of constant pressure and overwork can only continue at the cost of rising health problems and increasing numbers of people facing a warped and debilitating existence. A workplace needs to meet certain standards to be judged civilized. (Savage, 2006, p. 9)

Developing strategies to secure personal resilience is beneficial. If you are committing yourself to something that you believe will enhance your wellbeing and that is supported by sound evidence, then this is a reasonable action to take. If, however, the initiative is at the behest of your employer and stands within the context of an excessively demanding culture then it is also reasonable to challenge the motivation behind its introduction. It is important to be clear that someone is not offering you the equivalent of Coyote's steel helmet.

These ideas can help, together with other techniques outlined in this book. There are two important key ideas; firstly, build your resilience before it is needed and secondly remember Chris and how a quick fix was certainly not part of his story.

14

STRIKE A HAPPY MEDIA

If the only way you could read an email was to run a mile first, the urge would quickly die. Human beings constantly do subconscious effort/ reward calculations. Tapping a screen is the easiest of physical tasks.

(Weil, 2015)

In 2008, I wrote an unintended prequel to this book, *The Constant Leader*. One chapter was entitled *'Tool to Tyrant'* (pp. 57-61) and dealt with the overwhelm people were experiencing as they came to terms with a 24/7, connected work environment. It was packed with practical advice on managing the information flow and creating boundaries between us and this interconnected and free- flowing medium. The tenor of the chapter was that information exchange had changed up several gears and that we would have to adapt our existing practices in order to cope.

This is still a widespread even routine experience probably amplified by the increase in remote working. Since my attempts at handy hints for dealing with IT, I have increasingly moved from dealing with input to considering the impact of digital immersion. Fifteen years on, information technology has increased in both speed and capacity. The industry has created a growing number of platforms that have extended our engagement with digital devices and in turn changed the way that we engage with people and knowledge. My perspective is that our digital substrate is far less benign than we had previously thought. There is no suggestion that we become latter-day Luddites. I for one would not wish to return to that heady amalgam of the mechanical typewriter, Tipp-Ex and carbon paper or make international phone calls interrupted by an anxious parent gesticulating about the cost. However, as we fete ICT's Dr Jekyll, there is a need to reflect on his shadow alter-ego, Mr Hyde.

MR HYDE'S COMPUTER

Until recently, a visit to a high street betting shop would have brought you face-to-face with the 'Fixed Odds Betting Terminal' (FOBT). Introduced in 2001, these terminals allow players to bet on the outcome of various games with fixed odds, such as roulette. They raised astonishing amounts of revenue for their owners; in 2016, £1.8 billion pounds in the UK alone (Davies, 2017). Behind these takings is a string of tragic stories of individuals who have lost homes, families and jobs as they gambled as much as £100 every 20 seconds. Following campaigns to get them banned there was legislation brought in to limit their use. Davies (2020), writing in The Guardian, reviewed what was happening:

> High street bookies' £100-a-spin Fixed Odds Betting Terminals (FOBTs) became known as the "crack cocaine of gambling". They were linked to high rates of addiction and ruinous losses but produced massive profits. When the government limited their numbers to four per shop, the bookies opened more shops. Last year, after a long-running campaign, the

government reduced the maximum stake to £2. Some bookmakers sought to bypass the FOBT crackdown by quickly inventing new games that mimicked FOBTs while technically complying with the rules.

By now you are probably thinking that this argument has become somewhat tangential. However, the link lies in understanding the design of these machines and its relationship with the way that we interact with our own digital devices. FOBTs are skilfully designed using psychological insights to draw individuals into their maw. A *Guardian* editorial argues:

> FOBTs trade on a psychological insight: what keeps customers engaged is less the hope of winning than the pleasure of playing. They are designed to induce a state of 'flow', or being 'in the zone', in which all of the player's attention and consciousness is pulled into the game, and nothing from the outside world can impinge. It is, while it lasts, entirely satisfying. This is a similar mechanism to that which, in popular myth at least, leads teenagers, lost in their video games, to starve to death after playing for days and nights without sleep or food. It depends on speed of play, and infrequent but never predictable rewards. The knowledge that intermittent reinforcement works better than predictable rewards goes back to the psychologist BF Skinner's theory of conditioning, and the gaming industry takes full advantage of it. (*The Guardian*, 2017)

Underlying such fast and repetitive reward processes is the brain's dopamine system. In conditioning, the action is rewarded with the release of euphoria- inducing neurotransmitters, notably dopamine. The latter is released to encourage us to repeat life-sustaining activities such as eating healthy food, having sex, drinking water, and remaining in nurturing relationships. It is intended to operate within the context of healthy relationships and lifestyles. However, it can become detached and provide the springboard for developing damaging addictions such as overeating, drug and alcohol abuse, consumerism and, of course, gambling. So let us take a step back from the world of Paddy Power, Coral or Ladbrokes and return to our digital world. This same physiology drives our engagement with our laptops, smartphones and tablets. Many people routinely spread their attention across emails, texts, Instagram, Facebook, Pinterest, Snapchat, Twitter, Tik Tok and many others. It is not simply about choosing a social medium of choice but frequently trying for a blanket coverage across a number, perhaps as many as five or six.

If you are committed to maintaining a presence on social media then you will face two immediate pressures and a further potential one. Firstly, you will come under pressure to maintain the flow of your material and secondly your brain will become stimulated by an expectation of a response. While a lack of response can be disappointing, it is suggested that immediate or near-immediate responses can be more damaging. They position you squarely within the stimulus-response loop that is generating repetition by the release of dopamine. This really is not so far removed from the person enmeshed with gambling.

There is always the potential risk of adverse or critical comment which can be very damaging People can make abusive comments from an anonymous distance, levels of comment that they would never make in a face-to-face context.

It is not uncommon for people who are unable to access or

check their smartphones on a regular basis to display similar levels of stress as those seen in deprived smokers or drinkers. It is important to recognise that such behaviour is not about breaches of etiquette but it is actually evidence of dopamine-driven addictive behaviour.

The smartphone, our most portable digital device, is amazing in its capability and capacity. It can, of course, be used as a phone or to text, to calculate, to find addresses, access the internet, measure your exercise, get a weather forecast, track a friend, set your alarm, listen to music, diagnose medical conditions, construct to-do lists, play games etc. Its power exceeds mainframe computers in use even 30 years ago. It is almost impossible to compare one with Bletchley Park's Colossus Mk 2, built in 1944. This ran on 2,400 diode valves. In contrast, we can use our smartphone on the move and, because of its versatility, it will draw us into multitasking. We check Tik Tok whilst queuing, listen to music as we walk, connect to 24/7 rolling news as we eat and check what our friends are doing or saying even as we hold a face-to-face conversation with others.

Miller, a neuroscientist at the Massachusetts Institute of Technology, employs strong language when he refers to our alleged ability to multitask as a 'powerful and diabolical illusion'. One of the world's leading experts on divided attention, he states unequivocally:

> Our brains are not wired to multitask well ... When people think they're multitasking, they're just switching from one task to another very rapidly. And every time they do, there's a cognitive cost in doing so. (2013, p. 3)

He argues that we are not expert jugglers able to maintain a lot of balls in the air at once but, rather, that we are more like bad 'plate-spinners' rushing from one task to another and ignoring the one in front in order to give attention to others. This frantic activity is not the index of our productivity; in fact, the more diverse things that we do concurrently, the less efficient we become. Any form of multitasking will increase the level of the stress hormones cortisol and adrenaline in our bodies. Acting in tandem, these can overstimulate the brain and generate brain fog or disaggregate our thinking. Miller (2013), also argues that multitasking creates and sustains this dopamine-addiction feedback loop, which actually rewards the brain for losing focus. The prefrontal cortex is enchanted with the new and will easily allow the brain to redirect its focus and attention towards novelty. We are the ultimate cognitive jackdaws. Levitin, another neuroscientist, states:

> We answer the phone, look up something on the internet, check our email, send an SMS, and each of these things tweaks the novelty-seeking, reward-seeking centres of the brain, causing a burst of endogenous opioids (no wonder it feels so good!), all to the detriment of our staying on task. It is the ultimate empty-caloried brain candy. Instead of reaping the big rewards that come from sustained, focused effort, we instead reap empty rewards from completing a thousand little sugar-coated tasks. (2015, p. 1)

It gets worse. Ward *et al* (2017) found that cognitive capacity is significantly reduced when a person's smartphone is within reach, even if it is turned off. In their study, 800 smartphone users were asked to complete a series of tests on a computer. These were designed to require full concentration in order for an individual to achieve high scores. The tests were geared to measure participants' available cognitive capacity – the brain's ability to hold and process data at any given time. All participants were asked to turn their phones to silent. Some of the participants were randomly instructed to place their phones either next to them but face down, in a pocket or in a bag, while others were asked to leave their phones in another room.

The research project showed that where a participant had left their phone in another room, they significantly outperformed the group who had their phones on the desk beside them. They also, albeit slightly, outperformed those who had their phones in a pocket, briefcase or handbag. The findings suggest that the mere presence of our smartphone reduces our available cognitive capacity and impairs our cognitive functioning, even though we believe that we are giving the task in hand our full attention. When interviewed by Fotalia about his findings, Ward suggested that:

> As the smartphone becomes more noticeable, participants' available cognitive capacity decreases ... Your conscious mind isn't thinking about your smartphone, but that process – the process of requiring yourself to not think about something – uses up some of your limited cognitive resources. It's a brain drain. (2017, p. 1)

Ward and his team (2017) extended their reach in a further experiment. They looked at how an individual's self-assessed dependence on their smartphone mapped against cognitive capacity. The same series of computer-based tasks were used to assess performance. Again, participants were asked to switch their phones off and then randomly given similar locations to store them while the participants took the tests. The research findings indicated that the higher the level of dependency on the digital device of the participant, the worse the participant performed in the tests. However, putting the phone in an adjacent room restored the levels of their performance. The conclusion was that having your smartphone within sight or within easy reach reduces your ability to focus and perform tasks because part of your brain is actively working to ignore the phone.

PLAN TO THINK

This chapter appears to come out as 3-0 to the Luddites. Well perhaps not. It is clearly unreasonable to become a sort of IT version of King Canute. However, I would suggest that there is sufficient research to challenge or at least cause us to review our use of digital devices. Most of us engage with complex tasks both in our work and in our personal lives that require complex and certainly higher-order cognitive skills. Impairment, because we are being inhibited by the unregulated use of digital technology, cannot be argued as being likely to stack the odds in our favour when it comes to thinking things through.

So, five interventions to regulate your digital environment in order enhance your thinking:

- Use digital devices purposefully. Schedule times when you will be available to use them and do not let them become interwoven with real conversations or creative thinking. I worked for someone who is a red wine enthusiast. To keep his hobby in check he has followed the medical advice of having two days of abstention. Could this be a useful strategy to use with smartphones? Strangely, these abstinence days have never coincided with occasions when we have gone out for a meal.

- When undertaking complex tasks perhaps turn off your emails and leave your phone in another room. It is worth remembering that after being interrupted it can take about 25 minutes to get back to where you left off and that is after only a 2.8-second interruption. Error and tiredness are other negative consequences.
- Clear your bedroom of digital devices and remember their primary purpose. Leave your smartphone/tablet downstairs and do not use it as an alarm clock. In fact, buy a dedicated alarm clock with a switchable display, or even one with two bells on the top..
- Put a signature on your emails stating the times when you will be accessing them. *De facto*, this should include the weekends. That has certainly challenged me to think about my own stance on this issue.
- Consider reducing your presence on social media and reduce your time playing games.

High-quality thinking merits high-quality time that has as its hallmark a lack of interruption. Some will argue that this is an unreasonable expectation. The counter argument is that there is an unacceptably high cost to evolving organisations resulting from poorly structured leadership thinking.

THE METAVERSE

In many ways the Metaverse is the coming together of a number of components already being used in IT. The difference lies with the intensity of our interaction with a rising tide of artificial intelligence. It is immersive, proximal and interactive. The Metaverse will usually include us in a space of augmented reality and all virtual reality leading us to feel that we are in the

Internet itself. Angela Scanlon's recent TV show *Your Home Made Perfect* (BBC 2023) allows clients to experience architects suggestions for their home using virtual reality headsets. This kind of experience will become commonplace in medicine, education, design and virtual travel.

Technology is seldom neutral, explosives can be used in mining and at the same time provide an effective means to maim. There will be benefits which might well include mental, emotional and physical as the Metaverse is exploited. Conversely, negative side effects are almost inevitable. Potentially, digital alienation and addiction could add to the bonfire of growing mental health issues. Francis Haugen, a Facebook (Meta Platforms) whistle-blower, recently released hundreds of documents relating to social media platforms. In an interview she warned that the Metaverse will indeed be addictive (Scott 2022). Research by Hou et al (2019) has indicated that the internet, video games and social media in particular, can cause or exacerbate mental health issues such as anxiety or depression, and can be highly addictive.

Not surprisingly, the root of addiction and mental health centres in the brain with its stimulation of the regions of the brain responsible for pleasure by the neurotransmitters such as dopamine. With repetition, the brain and in turn the individual eventually begin to rely on that experience to feel good, and achieve their new normal state. A dependence has been built through this repetition and a narrow-focussed stimulation. This dependence, like all addictions is both physiological and psychological. Sternlicht, L. and Sternlicht A (2023) argue that:

> Video games release dopamine every time you advance towards the goal of the game, such as moving on to another level.

Social media releases dopamine every time you get a follow, like, comment or other engagement. Cryptocurrency trading and investing releases dopamine every time your investment increases in value or decreases if you are shorting the currency. When speculating on the Metaverse, everything seems to be what we currently experience in our digital world but on steroids. All virtual interactions are expected to be more intense and more stimulating, feeling much more real than what we currently experience through our phones, tablets and computers. In making an analogy to drugs, the Metaverse might be the fentanyl of heroin or the crack of cocaine; bringing about a more extreme and fast-acting high to the user. We can think of the impact this will have on virtual pornography addictions, virtual video game addictions, virtual social media addictions, virtual gambling addictions, etc. (p. 2)

Many others consider connection with others through Internet platforms to be the norm. Much working practice has changed to the point that it is deeply dependent on platforms such as Zoom and Teams. Separated families remain connected using these platforms. Social Media sites allow the sharing/ oversharing of personal information. Arguably, we are more connected, but it is important to recognise that it can impose a distance and drive us to be more alone and separated than ever. Many of the interactions occurring in the billions day by day lack authenticity and are not as satisfying as real-time relationships. Users of social media and its enhancement in the context of the Metaverse often believe that they are connecting with family and friends or creating new social circles whereas the reality is that they are in their own space and actually in most cases, alone. Gaming can leave the player isolated, connected by task and not relationship. Isolation also easily contributes to or exacerbates mental health issues which taken alongside the addictive dimension could pose a significant threat to our well-being and mental health. Real-time human engagement and authentic connection remains at the root of our humanity and the Metaverse is likely to be a poor substitute.

Powerful commercial interests may seek to reassure us that we are not heading towards a mental health apocalypse. Undoubtedly, there will be many positives which have the potential to enhance our lives. It is perhaps important to ask: are we embracing the technology or is the technology embracing us? There is a pressing need for research to bring clarity and protection before we find ourselves fumbling to try to force the genie back into the bottle.

15

SIMPLES

Two years ago, I bought a Land Rover. This is an iconic British vehicle which started life in 1947; mine was made in 1997. Its designer, Maurice Wilks, actually sketched out its design with a pointy stick in the sand on a beach on Anglesey. For reasons I am not entirely clear about, I had wanted one for some years. The vehicle had serious presence, sounded like a tractor and the roof leaked like a cheap umbrella.

Ownership brought me into a relationship with the local Land Rover specialists.

They were happy to guide me along the journey towards restoring Vera. Yes, I actually gave the vehicle a name! The discussions that I had with the enthusiastic proprietor took me to levels of detail that I had never imagined. The roof was white, but who knew there was so many shades available and that only one was correct for the respray. Every conversation and, in fact, most outings brought the possibilities of spending serious money on this geriatric vehicle.

It was bought on a whim, it was very much a fun car; my wife argued that the purchase redefined the term fun. Our 11 year-old grandson wanted to carry out a risk assessment before travelling in it. It was all too much, with Vera moving from a simple hobby towards me having a mechanical affair. I realised that this whole project was beginning to take up too much of my headspace. When I found my waking thoughts becoming filled with the task and the cost of the restoration of the vehicle it was time to rethink. Vera was found a new home on a farm. This comes close to the euphemism used by some parents to young children when they have the family pet put down.

Possessions are inevitable. Things become a significant part of our lives and conversations frequently include discussions about the malfunction of dishwashers, central heating systems, TVs and scams perpetrated on phones and laptops. One friend suffered real stress when the capsules in his new coffee machine kept exploding. He had to return it to the online retailer; suffice it to say that using a QR code in the local Post Office did not end well. I was in a meeting where the person leading it was clearly distracted. The previous day, she had decided to defrost her freezer and discovered that if you use a kitchen knife as your tool of choice, you can/probably will puncture the coolant carrying tubes and release the refrigerant gas into the atmosphere. The meeting soon developed a surreal quality as we discussed a key project, interspaced by phone conversations with a refrigeration engineer and a discussion as to whether to mend or replace the damaged appliance. The engineer's response was probably tinged with some reluctance as the damaged freezer was on the sixth floor of a block of flats. It was fascinating how this domestic mishap had grabbed a piece of my colleague's headspace and how much it derailed our meeting.

Each of our possessions and activities lays claim to a fraction of our head. In most cases, this is fairly small. On the other hand, the impact of some of our material possessions can be extremely intrusive. If you own an older car, just think for a moment how anxious you can become before the MOT; or alternatively, consider how stressed people become when their broadband fails. The more we own, then the more of our headspace has to be dedicated to funding their purchase, learning to use them, storing them, their maintenance and replacing them as they become obsolete or no longer state of the art or just worn out. We can come to a point where it begins to feel that our possessions are beginning to possess us.

As we assemble material possessions, clutter and just plain stuff, perhaps understanding the back story will help. Sweller (1988) is an Australian psychologist who has examined how we process information. His argument is that we have a long–term memory where we store the majority of our knowledge and experiences. It is analogous to storing data on a hard drive or Cloud storage. We also have a working memory where we engage in thinking and problem solving. Sweller's work is seen as significant and his extended thinking is not going to fit in a few short sentences here. One headline is that our working memory is quite small, usually cited as being between seven units of information plus or minus two units. So whilst extremely powerful and creative, it can readily come under strain if we start to use it like a fridge door with day-to-day information held by the mental equivalent of fridge magnets.

I was fascinated by a colleague's office. Every surface, including the floor, was covered with stacks of paper. There were curriculum materials, policy documents, correspondence, students' work and even various hobby-related magazines. It was spectacular, like the Manhattan skyline, modelled in print. Because he never threw anything away, he was always a good source for an elusive set of minutes or the departmental budget from five years earlier. It was intriguing how easily he could locate a document from what appeared to be a totally random pile. In the interest of transparency, I do need to confess that I also had a malicious desire to see one of these stacks collapse rather in the style of the latter phase of a game of Jenga.

His computer ran on similar principles with over 14000 emails in his inbox. His wallpaper picture of his family was obscured by huge numbers of documents stored on his desktop. Over time, my sense of awe at his ability to abstract information (and even his ability to walk from one side of his office to the other) faded. I realised that his amazing feats were inappropriate and that maintaining an index of the contents of his disordered lifestyle was using up a significant amount of his headspace.

LAGOM

This is a Swedish term that embodies a unique cultural philosophy and way of life. It's often translated to mean 'just the right amount' or 'engaging in moderation'. Perhaps its true essence goes much deeper and is rooted in the Swedish psyche; Lagom encapsulates the idea of balance simplicity and contentment.

The concept of Lagom extends to different aspects of life, from personal interactions, design and even governance. In social settings, he encourages inclusivity, equality, and consensus and intern promotes a harmonious community spirit. At work, it emphasises teamwork and cooperation, with everyone contributing to their fair share. In design and architecture, Lagom is evident in the minimalist yet functional and aesthetically pleasing approach.

Lagom encourages individuals to lead sustainable lives, avoiding excess and wastefulness. It encourages conscious consumption, reducing one's ecological footprint and respecting nature. In this sense, it aligns with the global movement toward sustainable living.

In the context of personal well-being, Lagom advises against extremes. It promotes a healthy work life balance, ensuring individuals have time for rest, leisure and relationships. He discourages overindulgence, some food, drink, or material possessions, advocating for self-control and gratitude for what one already has. The Swedish concept also ties into happiness and contentment. By avoiding excess and by not comparing oneself to others, individuals can find greater satisfaction with their own lives. Lagom fosters a sense of contentment with what is attainable and achievable, encouraging people to appreciate the present moment.

Overall, Lagom encapsulates a holistic and mindful approach to life, encouraging individuals to find equilibrium and happiness in simplicity and moderation. He continues to inspire people worldwide to embrace a more balanced and sustainable lifestyle. Brandmark (2017) suggests:

> By deliberately seeking a more manageable, comfortable, balanced way of doing things (I'm finding perfection in imperfection), you're taking the pressure off yourself – you're taking the pressures off others too. And you're gaining more of today's precious resource time. (page 110)

This chapter did not set out to advocate a philosophy of simplicity per se, though strong arguments can be made for living simply to reduce our impact on our planet. Rather, it is focussing on the benefits of decluttering our minds. I am suggesting that you collect and create strategies that allow you to unburden your cognitive systems and in turn reduce stress and boost our potential creativity.

GRI

I have deliberately set out a train of thinking departing from my mental station and I decided to cull my material possessions. This was not envisaged as being extreme, but rather more at the 'life's laundry' end of the spectrum. I implemented 'GR1' (Get Rid of 1 Thing Every Day). I recorded each item that I sold on Gumtree, gave away, took to a charity shop and even those that went to the tip. Some items were large, such as the two unwanted bikes that I sold; while some were small, like the read detective novel that went to the charity shop. Of course, it is important not to become obsessional or you will create a new preoccupation which would have the potential to eclipse the impact of the clutter and even leave you sitting on the floor.

I have done this for six months and it has been astonishing how much I have got rid of. This is about clutter and not essentials or memorabilia, it is not about becoming 'hair shirt' over possessions. However, alongside the obvious reduction in the unnecessary items that were filling my life, the process has felt quite cathartic. It has also reduced the casual purchase of further items. On mentioning GR1 to a few friends, some have decided to try it and their feedback has been unanimously positive.

The organisational writer Allen (2001) offers a rather stark conclusion. He also draws the analogy between the way the brain processes information and the RAM of a computer and argues:

> Everything you've told yourself you ought to do, your mind thinks you should do right now. Frankly, as soon as you have two things to do stored in your RAM, you've generated personal failure, because you can't do two things at the same time. This produces an all-pervasive stress factor whose source can't be pin-pointed. (2001, p. 23)

The head does not have a loft for the storage of clutter. Everything is present in one space, our headspace.

16

TOAST

My father was a talented engineer but there was a lack of skill transfer when it came to DIY projects. His signature method for making his toast was to use the grill and cook it until it was well done or what the rest of the family referred to as burnt. Installing the smoke detector on the kitchen ceiling had predictable consequences. When we visited, breakfast usually consisted of toast with an assault on the ears from the smoke alarm and a frantic and largely random flapping of a tea towel by him.

In a slightly tense conversation that followed one of these episodes, I outlined the options for moving to a calmer breakfast. My suggestions included moving the smoke alarm or restricting his diet to salads. Without saying a word, he handed me a screwdriver and left for a nearby café

So, a heart-warming, homespun metaphor which links nicely back to chapter 5 where trauma was considered. The similarity? In common with the inappropriately located alarm, memories around trauma are being stored in the wrong place. This happens as high levels of stress cause the hippocampus to begin to fail to handle memories and pass the role across to the amygdala; from archive to alarm centre.

So, can you relocate memories, and effectively sort out the filing system of your brain? Almost certainly not. Chapter 5 outlined how traumatic memories that were being stored in the amygdala can become a persistent present, rather than as a sepia toned album of our past. It was also mentioned that there were a number of techniques that had been used with military personnel with PTSD such as EFT and EMDR. This chapter will showcase EFT which is useful with trauma but also anxiety and depression.

It is rooted in the work of Callahan in 1979 where he developed Thought Field Therapy (TFT). It was argued that it had some links to acupuncture. Callahan applied it to PTSD, emotional problems and even cardiac arrhythmia. Devilly (2005) explored TFT and the then emergent EFT and other therapies including NLP. He concluded that there was no evidence for the claims made for these therapies and that they could even exhibit the characteristics of pseudoscience.

I had looked into EFT and had felt that some of the claims being made by practitioners were overblown and poorly substantiated claims were being made that serious diseases could be cured. A selection of variations including eye rolling and humming 'happy birthday' added to the essential tapping. Asking a client to hum happy birthday and roll their eyes sparked incredulity. At the time, I was very engaged in coach training for a large educational initiative in London, so I parked EFT, feeling both disappointed and perhaps even a little embarrassed about what I saw as some of the excesses.

Despite my reservations and usually when I had run out of possibilities, I did occasionally use it with clients. Each time, it produced results beyond anything that I had expected.

I worked with Joanne, an extremely able young lady, who worked in the financial services industry. When she came to make decisions, the residual influence from her mother ingrained from childhood was distorting the outcomes. It was almost as if she could hear her mother's voice in her head telling her what to do and what not to do, with an emphasis on the latter. I used EFT with outstanding results. She took hold of her career choices and almost immediately accepted a new post complete with a £30,000 salary increase. I was somewhat bewildered at the impact of the process and also left reflecting as to whether my fees were too low.

Gradually, a few supportive pieces of research began to emerge and these which have now become a flood. The Australian psychologists, Dr. Peta Stapleton and Dr. Dawson Church, have taken this research to another level. If you want to explore this further Stapleton (2022) has summarised much of the current research. In this context a headline perspective is probably appropriate.

Research has rules and these serve to take the research from opinion to something with substance. There are a core of EFT researchers, including the two mentioned above, who have sought to research and publish to high standards. This is both to understand the process but also to provide a rebuttal to some critics. There are a large number of public studies which are statistically significant. Many of them are randomised controlled trials around areas such as anxiety, depression and trauma. They have addressed the demands by the American Psychological Associations Division 12 task Force and the US government's National Registry of Evidence Based Programs and Practices. The latter imposes protocols for statistical procedures.

EFT has already been researched and more than 10 countries and by more than 60 investigators. Much of the work has been published in peer reviewed journals such as the *Journal of Clinical Psychology* and the *Journal of Nervous and Mental*

Disease. Gaining acceptance for EFT is not about conducting a war of attrition against detractors. However, every time research into the area is published in such journals then the efficacy, or indeed even its lack comes under considerable scrutiny.

Currently, EFT research is focused on replication of the key studies that have not yet been repeated. Further, contemporary research is exploring the changes in physiology that this deceptively simple technique induces using tools such as fMRIs, neurotransmitter analysis and latterly gene expression analysis.

There has also been a focus on meta-analyses, where randomised controlled trials are aggregated and the effectiveness of the treatment is reviewed statistically. This is expressed as a 'd' number (Cohen 1988). In the kind of analysis utilised a very small effect would come out as $d = 0.2$, a moderate outcome would be around $d = 0.5$ with a large effect coming in at $d = 0.8$. The effect size was found to be: PSTD $d = 1.23$ (Sebastian and Nelms 2016), anxiety $d = 1.23$ (Clond 2016) and depression $d=1.31$ (Nelms and Castel 2016). These are remarkable results which indicate an impact of EFT well outside the possibility of chance or placebo.

The research into EFT is extremely encouraging. It looks as if it is making a successful transition from being a bit niche to being accepted and used within mainstream medical practice. It is important to be upfront and not make specific claims as to its effective use. However, there do not seem to be adverse effects from its use, the dangers lie when an individual chooses to abandon existing medical advice such as prescription medications and adopt EFT as the replacement therapy. At the risk of being repetitive, that is definitely not being suggested.

HERE'S A STRAIGHTFORWARD GUIDE

This is contemporary EFT stripped to its essentials with no distractions.

1. Start by relaxing, letting thoughts go. Take some conscious breaths, in through the nose and then expire through the mouth. Bringing attention to a part of you that is connected to the floor e.g. feet or legs. Now start tapping your karate chop point firmly, just at a nice steady rate.
2. Notice the feeling(s), thought(s) memories that you would like to reduce. Locate the place in your body where you might experience these but keep tapping your karate chop point (the base of the little finger).
3. Score the intensity of the feeling, thought or memory from 0-10. 0 is non-existent and 10 is as bad as it can get.
4. Now label the thought/feeling/ memory with a short phrase or word. Trust what comes to mind as a label. If a label does not arise you can go with a phrase like 'these feelings' or 'these thoughts'.
5. Now, as you are tapping your karate chop point you create a set up phrase. Notice the first half is negative and the second part is affirming. These are examples of what a phrase might look like.

> Example 1: 'Even though I am anxious about making presentations, I completely love and accept myself.'
> Example 2: 'Even though I don't like confrontation, I completely love and accept myself.'
> Example 3: 'Even though I feel inferior to other people, I completely love and accept myself.'

6. the EFT process is carried out. You could even use your phrase and add at the end 'even if I do not'.

Once the 'set up' phrase is familiar, it is slowly repeated over and over as the EFT process is carried out. Keep tapping on the karate chop point as you repeat the phrase three times.

7. Then move to the sequence of points as follows, this time just using the label you chose (not the whole phrase) and say it 2-3 times on each tapping point (there is a diagram below to help):-
   - Inner edge of eyebrow
   - Outer edge of eye (on the bone)
   - Under the eye (on the bone)
   - Under nose
   - Under bottom lip
   - Collar bone lower edge – midway between shoulder and sternum
   - Under your arm
   - Over your heart/thymus point
   - Top of the head
8. Then move to your hand
   - Side of thumb
   - Side of first finger
   - Side of middle finger
   - Underside of little finger
9. Now take two conscious breaths.
10. Re score the thoughts/feelings
11. Re label them/it
12. Repeat the process until you take the score all the way to zero or an acceptable level to you in that moment.

The following diagram (Figure 16.1) will help you locate the tapping points. It is good to follow the sequence, but not slavishly. A mistake or two does not render the process invalid.

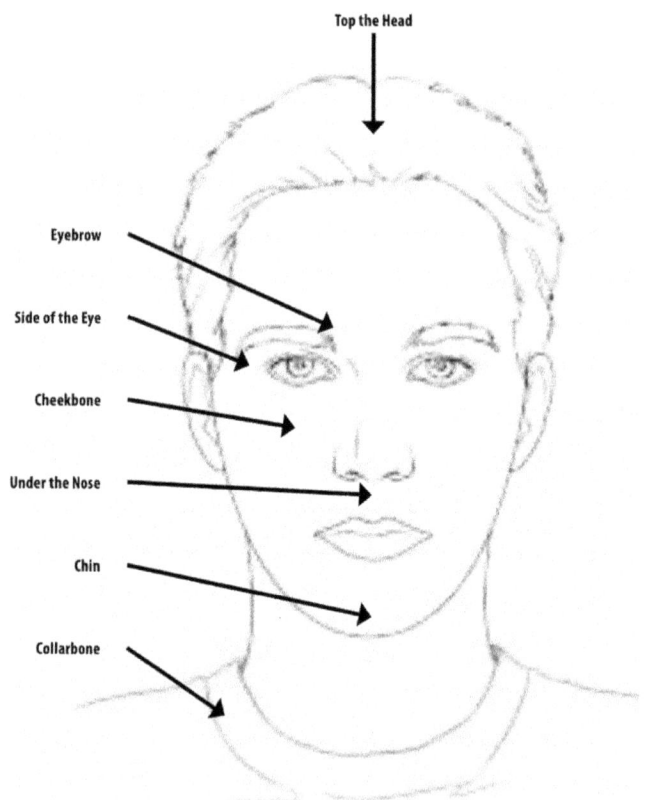

Fig. 16.1 EFT Tapping points

Use EFT several times a day for the first two weeks or so and you will find your brain gets used to it. It works by creating a "pattern interrupt", so called because it interrupts the over-regulation of your amygdala and resets it to a more normal and manageable level. Current research suggests that the benefits persist and that you do not have to keep topping up on a particular issue. This is well illustrated by the account at the end of the chapter.

Now you have the technique do not consign it to history. Keep extending your use of it to other areas of your life. This might include occasional pain, situations like a job interview or an exam where you are feeling nervous, or when feelings or thoughts come up that are not helpful to you.

JUST THINKING

Two years ago, I was admitted to hospital for investigations for a heart problem. I was told that the problem would be solved with having a stent inserted or possibly a couple. Further, that this would probably be day case surgery and with a holiday booked for the following week it came under my serious but not catastrophic category. Following the procedure, two doctors came to my bedside to discuss outcomes with me. Long faces and voices filled with professional concern framed my being told that they could not go the stent route and that the way ahead was having coronary bypass surgery in another hospital.

Maybe it was the disconnect with my expectations or even reading Bob Mortimer's (2021) comedic but graphic details of bypass surgery, but the doctors' words breached my defences. I was shaken; in the weeks that followed, I had repeated flashbacks to that conversation. With each replay of the memory, I felt the accompanying charged emotions as if they were freshly minted.

Two months later my friend Will Thomas rang. Incredibly supportive, he had just picked the wrong moment as I was on a twenty-minute break between doing two online doctoral supervisions.

Will asked me how I was getting on and I mentioned this intrusive and disturbing memory. He suggested doing some

EFT. I agreed, more out of politeness than dedication and I was more taken up with sorting my thoughts out before my next Zoom call. He took me through a couple of cycles of EFT. Despite being distracted by my work it worked. I repeated the cycle over the next couple of days and this traumatic memory was stripped of its power and persistence.

I have just had a tea break and revisited that hospital admission. Of course, I can remember the events, but the attendant alarming emotions are not there. This is nearly two years on.

17

ZEN AND THE ART OF SPOON CARVING

I was talking to my GP after that recent heart surgery. He asked what I was doing and my reply included the predictable such as taking moderate exercise and eating vegetables. Casually, I made mention of taking up spoon carving. He wanted to know if this involved sharp knives. He was not reassured when I replied 'Oh yes and an axe'. His view was that this might not be the hobby of choice for whom he had just prescribed anticoagulants. My comment that he would not have blood on his hands but that I might did not seem to lift the clinical mood.

It is accepted that spoon carving might not be for everyone. However, the focus involved in creating something that is recognizably spoon shaped (without amputation) is very relaxing. Other pressures and thoughts recede and my world becomes a redefined and much simpler space.

Of course, other crafts are available; painting, pottery, knitting, weaving, making jewellery and baking are all likely to achieve a similar effect. Often it seems that where there is a repetitive element, such as cycling away from traffic or walking and running, this works as well.

Before you embrace a craft there are other ways of 'knocking the brain out of gear'. When sleep was discussed, it was pointed out that the brain can still keep processing. In fact, excessive rumination will cause us to wake up. So, something more structured is often beneficial.

My train stopped at Clapham Junction. In itself, that was not a problem. Soon, an announcement was made that the train was delayed by a technical fault and that they were working to solve it as quickly as possible. From where I was sat, I could see an onboard computer monitor, and I watched with fascination as they switched the entire train operating system off and then on again.

It seemed to work, as we were soon moving again. The event generated a mixed response. On the one hand, I felt some satisfaction that they had used my method of choice when dealing with IT problems. I also felt some disquiet that this multimillion piece of technology was being sorted using the same low-tech approach. It set me wondering: should we use a similar approach with our brains? I concluded that employing a hard reset was probably not a great idea. Surely there are techniques that will reboot the brain without an intermediate phase of coma.

There will certainly be more than the three techniques that are considered in this book. EFT was explored in the previous chapter. Here two more are considered: mindfulness and 7/11 breathing. The former is a maintenance tool and the latter along with EFT are successful intervention strategies that can be used when we are stressed or dealing with invasive mind-sets.

Many of the surveys and statistics around mental health appear to have lagged behind. Some date back to 2014; however this would exclude the impact of the game changing pandemic. The following have been culled from a whole series of sources by The Priory Clinic (2021) and they seem to give a reasonable indication that action is very much needed:

- 1 in 6 people, or approximately 45.8 million adults, report experiencing symptoms for common mental health problems, like anxiety and depression, in any given week in England.
- Nearly half (43.4%) of adults (24.5 million in England) think that they have had a diagnosable mental health condition at some point in their life.
- 61% of adults with mental health conditions don't access treatment.
- The amount of people with common mental health problems went up by 20% between 1993 to 2014, in both men and women.
- 14.3% of deaths worldwide, or approximately 8 million deaths each year, are attributable to mental disorders.
- 98% of people agree that mentally ill people experience stigma and discrimination.
- Nearly 9 out of 10 people with mental health problems say that stigma and discrimination have a negative effect on their lives.
- 25% of people in England, approximately 14.1 million adults, say they feel lonely at least some of the time.

Many of these statistics would benefit from a greater level of detail. They do show mental health issues to be pervasive and serious. The response in the UK gives every indication of being stretched well beyond its capacity to provide appropriate support:

> At the same time, 45% reported a fall in routine appointments, suggesting that self-isolation, shielding, school closures, and fear of engaging with health services because of the risk of infection may be keeping patients away.

Wendy Burn, president of the Royal College of Psychiatrists, said, "We are already seeing the devastating impact of covid-19 on mental health with more people in crisis. But we are just as worried about the people who need help now but aren't getting it. Our fear is that the lockdown is storing up problems which could then lead to a tsunami of referrals. (Torgeson 2020, p. 369)

It is the argument of this book that it is as important, if not more important, to develop strategies to avoid these distressing and often dark conditions. This is especially true for mindfulness. Its regular use will help secure positive mental health. That cliché, 'If it ain't broke, don't fix it', may apply to your lawnmower but it definitely does not apply to your head.

MINDFULNESS

Mindfulness has its origins in Buddhism and for a number of years was seen as being somewhat alternative. It has now moved centre stage and is being widely advocated and has become increasingly mainstream. The following quotation is from the NHS Choices website (2017):

> Mindfulness is recommended by the National Institute for Health and Care Excellence (NICE 2017) to way to prevent depression in people who have had three or more bouts of depression in the past. There are a growing number of studies that support its use and effectiveness with anxiety and depression e.g. Branstrom et al (2011) and Bayer et al (2008).

Human beings are unique in the animal kingdom in that they can reflect or even ruminate on the past and also speculate on what might happen in the future. Poor mental health and even poor performance can often be traced to spending too much time in those spaces where we have little or no agency. The more the pressure mounts, the more we try to explain how we have got into this particular position and then make predictions about the future which are quite likely to move to the apocalyptic end of the prophetic spectrum. Mindfulness is about returning us to the present and using techniques to drag us away from rumination and unlikely futures. Imagine that you are driving a car up a long and very steep gradient and the engine starts to overheat. The best strategy is to pull off the road, put the car into neutral and let it idle until it cools own.

Mindfulness does much more than let the overheated individual return to an appropriate operating temperature. It also changes the way in which the very circumstances that they are dealing with are viewed. Regular engagement with mindfulness gives us this changed perspective as an enduring legacy.

The information on mindfulness is legion: web-based courses, phone apps, books, face-to-face courses and personal training. My suggestion is that you start both simply and with a commitment to incorporating it in your daily routine. Begin with as little as five minutes in the morning and then perhaps build up to two sessions each day and perhaps eventually extend these sessions to 20 minutes. I also incorporate mindfulness into other daily activities such as eating (where I slow down and savour each mouthful) and walking the dog (where I take notice of my surroundings, from the macro to the micro). I even drink tea mindfully!

Faced with this level of time commitment, many already stressed and pressured people will dismiss the idea as great in principle but unconnected to the time demands that they are under. The simple response is that no athlete neglects effective preparation. 'Just Do It' is seldom a great platform of choice.

Meditation lies at the core of mindfulness and the following exercise is a great place to start and will certainly pay tangible dividends. It works best in a quiet place where you will not be disturbed. You will need an upright but comfortable chair.

Stage 1 (60 Seconds)
Breathe purposefully
Sit in the chair in an upright position with the small of your back pressed against the back of the chair. With your feet flat on the floor, place your hands in a comfortable position on your thighs. Close your eyes or let them look forward in an unfocused way. For a moment, just notice how your feet feel on the floor; it might be hard or soft. Begin to breathe purposefully, either through the nose or the mouth. Consciously breathe in and then exhale more slowly. (See the later section on 7/11 Breathing) Keep going for approximately one minute.

Stage 2 (60 Seconds)
Move at your own pace
Now, stop counting and let your breathing settle into a pace that feels natural to you. Pay attention to what each breath feels like; compare your rhythm of breathing with how you normally breathe. Observe how the breaths are formed as they start with the abdomen and then move upwards to the shoulders.

Stage 3 (60 Seconds)
Retain your focus
Continue to be aware of your breathing and this natural cadence that you have adopted. Usually, at this stage, thoughts and ideas

will start to intrude; 'to do lists', appointments, challenging issues, perhaps even problem people. Do not try to exclude them or allow them to become a dominating focus. Instead, start to visualise them as a being like a cloud floating past, observed but harmless. Visualising issues in this way will allow you to acknowledge your concerns without becoming emotionally overwhelmed by them. If a thought does not drift away, it is often helpful to make a note of it on a notepad and return to your meditation.

Stage 4 (60 Seconds)
Relax
You have been focusing on your breathing. Now, simply sit, reminding yourself that there is nothing you are required to do at this time.

Stage 5 (60 Seconds)
Gratitude
Finally, call to mind something that you are grateful for. It may be a relationship, a beautiful day, improved health or even just the chance to spend some time meditating.

Connect with your body, noticing how relaxed your muscles are, the steady rhythm of your heart. If your eyes have been closed, open them. Stand up and move forward with the rest of your day in a calm and resourceful state.

Table 16. 1 (Adapted from the 'Five-Minute Meditation', Liao, 2017)

Engaging with mindfulness is not a luxury, but an essential: it increases concentration by reducing stress; it increases our range of options when we are making decisions; and it improves engagement with people by transferring attention from ourselves to them. Luders *et al* (2012) even found that this kind of meditation changes neural structure. Their work suggests that it will increase the amount of gyrification of the brain – that is, the folding of the cortex tissue on the outside of the brain. This actually allows the brain to process information faster.

7/11 BREATHING

This is very much a 'break the glass in case of emergency' technique. Our breathing is on autopilot for most of the time. Probably, until you read this chapter, you had not even thought about whether you were breathing or not. Unusually for a physiological function, we can take back control and regulate our breathing rate or even hold our breath.

If you purposefully breathe out longer than you breathe in, your body will calm down. This response to slowing down your breathing rate is inevitable, it is hardwired into your nervous system; there's simply no way round it for your body. Shallow rapid breathing is very much part of the stress scenario and should be avoided. The 7/11 breathing technique simply puts some structure into how we can regulate our breathing.

If you start to feel anxious or stressed:

1. Pause.
2. Focus on your breathing.
3. Breathe in through your nose to the count of 7.
4. Breathe out slowly through your mouth to the count of 11.

In a minute or so, you will have calmed down to a surprising degree. Crucially, it is about breathing slowly and deliberately and maintaining the ratio of the times that you inhale and exhale.

Weil (2015) demonstrates a variation of this technique. He advocates breathing in to the count of 4, holding whist counting to 7 and exhaling through the mouth for the count of 8. This method seems to work particularly well for getting off to sleep.

Threat activates our fight-or-flight response and stimulates the sympathetic nervous system, getting us ready for action. The parasympathetic nervous system works in the opposite manner and moves us to a bodily state of rest or relaxation. It is the out-breaths that bring this system into play. When you are startled, you will often take a sharp intake of breath. However, after a good meal you might move your chair back from the table and sigh deeply: an out-breath. Not surprisingly, a breathing technique with longer out-breaths than in-breaths will be more effective at lowering emotional arousal and it is resonant with us achieving a naturally relaxed bodily and mental state.

OUT OF SIGHT, OUT OF MINDFULNESS

Mindfulness isn't difficult. We just need to remember to do it. (Salzberg, 2010, p. 17)

The quotation at the opening of the chapter is from one of the pioneers in the current wave of meditation and mindfulness, Sharon Salzberg. She hits the nail squarely on the head when she argues for its routine use. Mindfulness, in particular, is being taught in schools and many commercial settings. It is burgeoning in professional development days. I regularly advocate its use with my clients. Often, they respond with something to the effect of 'I know all about this. We had a day on it.' Initially, I was encouraged to hear this but my optimism was soon dispelled as it became evident that their knowledge and practice were not in the same room.

These deceptively simple techniques connect with our physiology and psychological processes in profoundly beneficial ways. They must, however, be applied with a degree of persistence if they are to work. The argument has been made that anxiety and stress are either hardwired into our brains or else we have learnt negative patterns of behaviour and thinking, such as catastrophisation. Changing these is completely possible, but it is unreasonable to expect the process of change to be passive.

I am concluding with a story that certainly has its origins way back in history. I came across is from Tyrell (2015):

Once, a beautiful princess sat by an ornate pool in her palace grounds. As she peered down, admiring her beautiful reflection on the surface of the clear pool, her priceless crown suddenly slipped from her head and into the waters with a splash.

She screamed for her attendants to retrieve her precious crown and they leapt into the waters, frantically searching, scrabbling around, a flurry of activity. But all this effort merely brought up mud and debris from the bottom of the pool, making it even harder to find the missing crown...

Eventually, an old storyteller arrived on the scene. He began to tell such a riveting tale of times gone by that, despite themselves, all the princess's aides stopped searching and relaxed. Even the princess momentarily forgot about the missing crown and listened to the man's sweet words. By the time he'd finished telling his tale, not only had everyone calmed down, but the mud from the pool had settled and the waters were again clear.

At that point, the storyteller reached down into the water and retrieved the princess's crown, which could now clearly be seen. (Tyrrell, 2015, pp. 45-46)

Like most metaphorical stories, it can be explored and applied in different ways. However, in this context it provides an excellent insight into the way persistent mindfulness is so relevant in allowing our minds to clear and support our thinking and of decision-making in particular. The cognitive mud settles and mental clarity is secured.

18

THE RELENTLESS PURSUIT OF PEACE

I had a conversation with a friend whose car has been off the road for nearly two months. A small microswitch, under the brake pedal, had failed and it was linked to the automatic transmission of the car. He outlined the problem as: sometimes the car will not start and sometimes I cannot turn it off. I would readily concede that neither of these options are good.

The failure of this small electrical component had rendered his two-ton SUV unpredictable and created a significant source of personal stress as he was without transport. A car is an amalgam of around 30,000 parts. This level of complexity pales into insignificance alongside that of our brains. Our brains are the last and grandest biological frontier, and the most complex thing we have yet discovered in our universe. Each brain contains around 86 billion neurones interlinked through trillions of connections. My guess is that at some point something is going to go wrong. There could be damage through injury, deterioration through disease or aging, perhaps even the incredible processing power can become overwhelmed by our circumstances.

The message of this book is that whilst our brains are not the whole story of who we are, they are centre stage in framing our identity, intentions and their expression. To support our brain's function and our wellbeing it deserves more than an occasional spa day or a couple of paracetamol.

In this legacy chapter, it is useful to reiterate a key focus. Underpinning so much of what has been written is the relentless pursuit of peace. It is this peace rather than the more vacuous happiness that can confront mental health malfunction, stress, depression and anxiety. It is peace that provides an antidote to depression. Powerful tools that support the achievement of peace have been outlined in previous chapters such as mindfulness and EFT. The review and reordering of how we live has been explored. It would be unrealistic to suggest that we can sidestep every problem or stress grenade, but we must keep centring on peace.

Writing this book has been a challenge because throughout, my own life has continued with a particular intensity. At each point and turn I have had to take stock of my thinking and my own words and apply them to my personal circumstances. Sometimes, this has been successful and sometimes I have got it wrong and had a bit of a wallow in self-pity or gone up the stress Richter scale.

The last two months have been a case in point. I had a mole removed from my back and was given assurances that it was almost certainly OK. The 'almost' qualification has lingered in the shadows as I waited for the delayed histology results. Three purely social conversations, just catch ups, suddenly went into very dark places as friends talked about their suicidal thoughts. I hate the thought of their distress but I also started to mentally churn about whether what I had said to them was appropriate. I just did not see those conversations coming. My eldest son, very much an adult, has stayed with us and discussed how to move his career forward. He decided to alleviate his own stress by doing some woodturning on my lathe. He has a grip like a gorilla on a testosterone supplement. A key solid steel component fractured, and I have had to try and source a replacement. My wife loves childcare, and circumstances have meant a bonus dose of our young grandchildren. Whilst they are lovely, they are still a presence. I had to write a presentation on mental health and crafting, whilst stimulating to write, you would have to ask the audience about the quality of the delivery. A persistent cough has led to disturbed sleep. I wrote a paper on a controversial topic that was well received by some and not well received by others. Suffice it to say that the readership of this article did not hold back. I had to dredge the material being produced by Jordan Peterson in order to support a relative. Our dog injured his leg. The list goes on with a backing track of the Ukrainian war, inflation, the failure of the Silicon Valley Bank, the absence of vegetables in the supermarkets, the problems of the NHS and a smorgasbord of national strikes. One morning I woke up and described myself as 'bumping along the bottom', in other words having a low mood. Actually, what did I expect was going to happen; my own model of the brain was coming in right on cue.

Time for some serious and immediate action. I got going on the EFT around the anxiety about my mole. I made sure that I scheduled in mindfulness. Took a break from our childcare. Reframed my crafting presentation as being a fascinating day listening to others rather than being a presentational pit that I had become convinced that I was going to fall into. Stopped walking the dog for a few days. Ditched Jordan Petersen and moved to watching *Countryfile* and *The Repair Shop*. Stopped the watching of rolling news and bought some *Fisherman's Friends* cough sweets (other brands are available).

Not all the things impact us equally. It would be facile to equate the damage to my woodworking lathe with Putin's aggressive war in the Ukraine. There is, however, a flaw in this argument. We can apply some index of severity to some of the things that are going on in our lives. This is absolutely right for an imminent and threatening problem like friends talking about suicide. However, for many of the issues in our lives our heads are a 'one stop shop' with problems taking up headspace and adding quantity which is not always about the particular problem's severity. Sometimes, we are just spinning too many plates. Whatever we can change or confront will have a significant impact on the way that we feel. There is a need to prioritise around immediate threat but perhaps not always get too taken up with ranking our problems to the distraction of recognising their number.

Will Thomas, who gets a number of name checks in this book, but sadly no share of the royalties, gave me these *Serenity Questions:*

- What can I control? (my own mind, ideas, perspective, my inner world)
- What can I influence? (this could be ideas, systems, other people, it is very much linked to where you put your energy and about not wasting it on projects which do not have traction)
- What might I need to come to accept? (be at peace with; it is not defeat to accept things which you cannot control – I have a friend who is still railing about decimalization – that ship sailed in 1971!)

These are an extremely useful framework to examine what we are thinking and doing. Putting issues in the wrong category is extremely counter-productive as we try to control situations that are beyond our reach. Sometimes, there are past events that it is simply time to archive.

FLASHES OF BRILLIANCE

Peace is not just to go to state when we feel overwhelmed, stressed and beginning to drop the ball. It is also the home of creativity and sometimes it is so powerful a state that great ideas can be born in a moment and in unusual places. One of the most famous accounts of a 'flash of brilliance' concerns the 19th century chemist, August Kekule.

A staple of organic chemistry that has led to the development of plastics, pharmaceuticals and supported our study of physiology is the way that the element carbon can provide a skeleton for very complex chemicals such as DNA. One problem that has challenged chemists for a number of years was how the element carbon bonded to form rings, as in the case of the compound benzene. Kekule proposed the theory as to how this took place and intern facilitated the development of a whole new branch of organic chemistry. This was extremely important for both pure and applied chemistry. In 1980, 25 years after his discovery, he was honoured by the German chemical society (Verderese and Roth, 2011). Kekule spoke at this meeting of how he derived his ground-breaking theory. He related that he had discovered the ring shape of the benzene molecule after having a daydream. This dream included visualising an ancient symbol known as the Ouroboros which depicts a snake or serpent eating its own tail. He suggested that this vision was rooted in his long-term study of the nature of carbon-carbon bonds.

There is a long line of such discoveries: Archimedes leaping from his bath and developing the idea of specific gravity; Sir Timothy Berners-Lee's conceptualisation of the world wide web; Sir Alexander Fleming's discovery of penicillin; and even Albert Einstein's theory of relativity, which bizarrely he conceived whilst riding a bike. These are inspirational stories, though some are mired in urban mythology. However, what does become clear is that significant creative thinking often happens as 'flashes of brilliance'. Of course, the execution of these ideas can then take considerable effort and planning.

Back in 2011 a group of us were conducting research into the experiences of newly appointed headteachers working in urban environments (Earley et al 2011). I undertook some of the field research and interviewed a number of these headteachers who contributed to our study. They spoke of how they often came up with solutions to difficult problems when they were doing repetitive tasks. They mentioned cycling, running and even being in the shower as providing seminal moments for coming up with solutions to problems that they had seen as being extremely challenging. These tasks were somehow facilitated as much of their mind and body moved into autopilot. Even this book (and here I open myself up to potential criticism) was originally conceived both in terms of its overall theme and even some of its content while driving home late one night between the Fleet and Winchester services on the M3 motorway.

THE MIDNIGHT MILKMAN

As a teenager, I lived in a small Staffordshire village which was over a mile from the main road and only had two buses a week. I was the first pupil to go to the grammar school, some five miles away, for many years. Unremarkable, except that children in the village used to throw stones at me as I cycled home in my uniform.

We had a local milkman, always referred to as Mr Cartwright. He was an institution, getting his deliveries through whatever the weather. However, it was debatable whether a particular drop-off was early for tomorrow or late for yesterday. Eventually, even our dog stop barking at rattling milk bottles at two in the morning

Mr Cartwright modelled depression; as he walked, his head was bowed under his trilby and the Rudolph nose provided a testimony to his heavy drinking. He seldom spoke. My mother had a constant challenge to pay this nocturnal tradesman. One of our neighbours had been unable to find him and pay him for over six months; this must have strained his somewhat tenuous cash flow.

He was part of village life, a character and whilst there were numbers of other locals vying for his coveted idiosyncrasy award, he held on to it for many years. It was after his death that the tragedy of his life came to light. As a young man, he had become an unintentional father and in the expectations of the time he had married. His wife was very much in the style of Kathryn in The Taming of the Shrew, though he had been less successful. Even as a teenager, I could see that he was treated with contempt by his family and many of his customers. Less well-known was that he had started life as a concert pianist and that his change of circumstances had dictated a very different pathway from the one that he had originally set out on. Subsequently, drink became a mental analgesic. After his premature death, his dilapidated cottage was sold to developers. The demolition providing a tragic epitaph for his unfulfilled life as they pulled the cottage down around a neglected baby grand piano. This was a final act showing that his considerable skill had found no appreciation from those around him.

It is strange how stories from years ago can surface in our minds; perhaps that is just an age thing. Mr Cartwright came to my mind quite vividly as I started to explore the Japanese concept of Ikigai. I do accept that connecting a Staffordshire milkman with a Japanese lifestyle tool is a bit of a jump. Ikigai was described by Kumano

(2018) as a feeling of accomplishment and fulfilment that usually follows when people pursue their passions. The feeling of Ikigai is generated when we undertake activities that are not imposed on us; they are often spontaneous and undertaken willingly and our personal actions are very much linked to our inner self.

The following diagram is often used a summary of Ikigai. It is a bit like a compass with four points, though unlike a compass, we have to explore our direction of travel to each of the points simultaneously:

- What I love to do
- What the world needs
- What I get paid for
- What I am good at

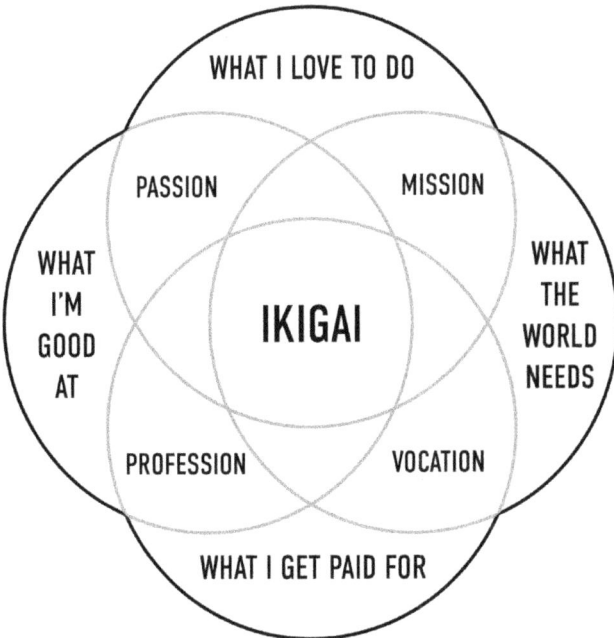

Fig. 18.2 An outline of Ikigai

Our Midnight Milkman became detached from his music; the thing that he was passionate about and which provided opportunities to experience self-efficacy had gone with that. I suppose that in performing he had brought joy to others and he had been deprived of that. Probably his budget had collapsed under his depression driven business style. It is easy to see how he had been stripped of fulfilment and become the antithesis of a life well-lived. Not everybody models an Ikigai collapse in such a sustained and toxic manner. Many people do get the balance wrong and pay for being out of kilter with a diminished sense of happiness and fulfilment.

Consider for a moment the *what I get paid for/financial needs* dimension. Most of us need to work in order to earn a living. It may be that our job is absolutely something we are good at and that we derive huge satisfaction from work that is far from the daily grind. It is simply not what we want to do. You will have heard that story from vets, doctors, teachers and even stand-up comedians. Earning has come to dominate their world and eclipsed the other areas of Ikigai. Money and status can easily become entangled with ownership of premium items like watches, cars or having a self-indulgent lifestyle as these become seen as being an entitlement. We can become seduced by our consumer society and our needs for material acquisition demanding to be satiated. A good income is valued by most of us, but surely not one that has to service excessive spending or debt? It is perhaps worth visiting re-visiting *Chapter 14 – Simples* and reflecting on the tipping point between our needs and wants.

I was speaking with a friend who is a medical physicist. Highly skilled, but unable to work to his personal satisfaction because of an excessive workload. At a stroke, he felt his sense of professionalism was downgraded. He subsequently made some adjustments to his lifestyle and is engaging in wildlife photography. The latter was bringing enjoyment and a sense of self-efficacy. He is also a member of his local church where his musical skills are very much appreciated. Despite these offsetting his needs, these activities will probably not sufficiently counterbalance the deficit being experienced in his job. Probably, some level of change of career will have to be negotiated.

One more example to emphasise just how interconnected the model is. Consider for a moment, the *what the world needs/altruism* strand. Imagine that you have volunteered to work in a food bank, an organisation which has sadly become so important in these challenging economic times. It is volunteering; so you will not get paid which knocks that strand out, and you will probably have to fund your own travel expenses. You have been allocated the task of sorting produce into bags, tedious but necessary. However, your own background is in marketing and your offers to help with publicity have been ignored and you are still putting pasta into bags. This is definitely not touching the *what I'm good at/self-efficacy* aspect. There is that final strand, *what I love to do/fulfilment* one. You are a compassionate person and so the food bank connects with this. However, part of your compassion engages with your enjoyment of having conversations with other people. Your back office role is not coming together in a way that is supporting your needs and now your motivation is beginning to flag. It is probably time to renegotiate your role or set a time limit on how long you will continue with the bags. It is not unreasonable to accept that whilst you want to help this might not be the organisation for you and find another outlet for your altruism.

Ikigai is a useful tool to take stock of our lives and examine our work/life balance. There is also the model which was considered as at the start of this book, Fig. 2.1.

THE STRUCTURE OF
— MENTAL HEALTH —

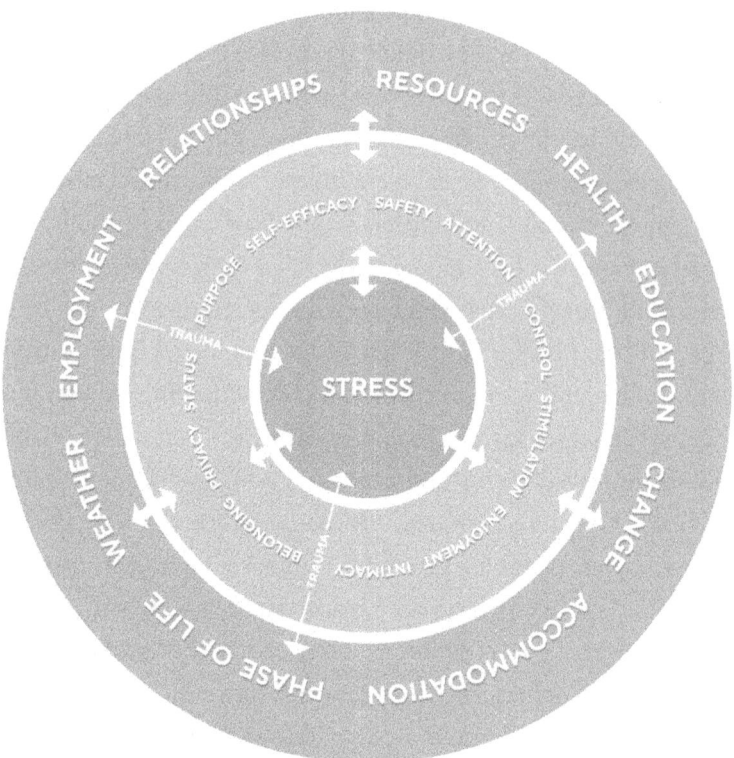

Fig. 2.1. The structure of mental health

THE CLOCK

Imagine owning a beautiful long-case clock or a bracket clock, probably fronted by an ornate dial. You could just use it to tell the time, or you could become fascinated by the highly crafted workings. Using the clock just as a time piece is fine. Becoming totally absorbed by the mechanism and, possibly the history of manufacture, misses the point. In a similar way, you could simply use this book to make changes and engage in your own relentless pursuit of peace. Some people might mine the book for information and miss out on the opportunity for personal transformation. It might be that you have reached the last chapter and are concerned that what you have read might lack substance, just another self-help book that is characteristically ephemeral. For the latter reader, I have sought to reveal the mechanism behind the clock face and refer the ideas and research back to source, perhaps tedious but it is there.

Will it work? Absolutely, but like many things in life, only if it is used as directed. Some techniques like EFT have a life gripping persistence that often does not need reinforcement. Other approaches like mindfulness or gratitude have a diminished impact if they are not used routinely. Flossing was never intended just for the evening before your dental appointment.

Our personal context will frequently erode our peace, even our mental health and wellbeing. Few of us live without the intermittent spectre of destructive challenge being close. Many of us may need to make changes to our context. All of us, however, need to pursue peace with a relentless tenacity. This is not because it is fashionable or loosely beneficial but because it is essential to our wellbeing, happiness, fulfilment, health and engaging with our potential.

References

Adams, R., Boscarino, J. and Figley, C. (2006) Compassion Fatigue and Psychological Distress Among Social Workers: A Validation Study. *Am. J. Orthopsychiatry.* 2006 Jan; 76(1): 103-108.

Allen, D. (2001) *Getting things done.* London: Piatkus.

American Psychiatric Association (2013) *Diagnostic and Statistical Manual of Mental Disorders, 5th Edition (DSM-5.* Washington DC: American Psychiatric Association.

Ariely, D., Gneezy, U., ; Loewenstein, G., and Mazar, N. (2005) *Large stakes and big mistakes,* Boston MA: Federal Reserve Bank.

Ashraf, A. and Nassar, S. (2018). "American Muslims and vicarious trauma: An explanatory concurrent mixed-methods study". *American Journal of Orthopsychiatry.* 88 (5): 516–528.

BBC (2017 – present) *The Repair Shop.* London: BBC.

BBC (1988 to present) Countryfile. London: BBC.

BBC (2023) *Your Home Made Perfect.* London; BBC.

Bandura, A. (1963) *Social learning and personality development.* New York: Holt, Rinehart, and Winston.

Barratt, A.(2006) *Resource Review.* Available at: https://ebm.bmj.com/content/ebmed/11/3/93.full.pdf (Accessed 22nd February 2023).

Barrett, L., (2020) *Seven and a Half Lessons About the Brain.* London: Picador.

Beyerstein, B. (1999). Whence Cometh the Myth that We Only

Use 10% of our Brains? In Sergio Della Sala (ed.). *Mind Myths: Exploring Popular Assumptions About the Mind and Brain*. New Jersey, Wiley.

Bowden, M. (2013) *Tame the Primitive Brain: 28 Ways in 28 Days to Manage the Most Impulsive Behaviors at Work.* New Jersey: John Wiley & Sons Inc.

Brantmark, N (2017) *Lagom, the Swedish Art of Living a Balanced, Happy Life*. London: Harper Collins.

Bremner, J. (2006) Traumatic stress: effects on the brain. *Dialogues Clinical Neuroscience* 2006 Dec; 8(4): 445–461.

Brontë, C. (1847) *Jane Eyre*. London: Smith, Elder & Co.

Carroll, L. (2014) *Alice's adventures in Wonderland*. London: Macmillan Children's Classics. .

Clond M. Emotional Freedom Techniques for Anxiety: A Systematic Review With Meta-analysis. J Nerv Ment Dis. 2016 May;204(5):388-95.

Coates, M. (2008) *The Constant Leader*. London: Network Continuum.

Coates, M (2018) *It's Doing My Head In*. Ipswich: John Catt Educational.

Coates, M. and Bingham, D (2020) Putting a Sticking Plaster on a Gaping Wound – Exploring the Provision Being Made in English Secondary Schools to Support Mental Health and Mental Well-Being . *Buckingham Journal of Education* 2020; 1: 149 – 177.

Coates, M. (2022) The Blind Wood Turner. *Beyond Education that Counts*. Available on: https://anchor.fm/beyondeducation. (Accessed 5th March 2023).

Cohen, J. (1988). Statistical Power Analysis for the Behavioral Sciences (2nd ed.). Hillsdale, NJ: Lawrence Erlbaum Associates, Publishers.

Craft, L. and Perna, F. (2004) 'The benefits of exercise for the clinically depressed', *Primary Care - Companion to The Journal of Clinical Psychiatry* 6 (3) pp. 104-111.

Crockett, M. J., Siegel, J. Z., Kurth-Nelson, Z., Ousdal, O. T., Story, G., Frieband, C., Grosse- Rueskamp, J. M., Dayan, P. and Dolan, R. J. (2015) 'Dissociable effects of serotonin and dopamine on the valuation of harm in moral decision making', *Current Biology* 25 (14) pp. 1852-1859.

Crawford, A. and Bell, B. (2022) *Molly Russell inquest: Father makes social media plea.* BBC 1st October 2022. Available at: https://www.bbc.co.uk/news/uk-england-london-63073489. (Accessed 3rd October 2022)

Csikszentmihalyi, M. (1990). *Flow: the psychology of optimal experience.* New York, NY: Harper & Row.

Davies, R. (2020) How Britain Got the Gambling Bug , *The Guardian*, 16th January 2020. Available at: https://www.theguardian.com/society/2020/jan/16/how-britain-got-the-gambling-bug.

Deci, E. L., & Ryan, R. M. (1985). *Intrinsic motivation and self-determination in human behaviour.* New York: Plenum.

Denning, S. (2007) *The Secret Language of Leadership.* San Francisco; Jossey-Bass.

Denning, S. (2011) *The leader's guide to storytelling.* San Francisco, CA: Jossey-Bass.

Devilly, G. (2005) Power therapies and possible threats to the science of psychology and psychiatry. *Australian & New Zealand Journal of Psychiatry.* 39 (11), pp. 437–445.

Dickens, C. (1843) *A Christmas Carol.* London: Chapman and Hall.

Dijk, D., Groeger, J. A., Stanley, N. and Deacon, S. (2010) 'Age-related reduction in daytime sleep propensity and nocturnal slow wave sleep', *Sleep* 33 (2) pp. 211-223.

Dijksterhuis, A & van Knippenberg, (1998) *The Relation Between perception and Behaviour, or How to Win a game of trivial Pursuit*, Journal of Personality and Social psychology Vol. 69, No. 5.

Dundurn (?), (2008) Leadership and Lack of Moral Fibre in Bomber Command, 1939–1945: Lessons for today and tomorrow", (2008) in Coombs, Howard (ed.), *The Insubordinate and the Noncompliant: Case Studies of Canadian Mutiny and Disobedience, 1920 to Present*, p. 101–204.

Earley, P., Nelson, R, Higham, R., Bubb, S., Porritt, V., Coates, M. (2011) Experiences of new headteachers in cities. Nottingham, NCSL.

Elliott, R. and Tyrell, M. (2002) *The depression learning path*. Oban: Uncommon Knowledge.

Epstein, R. (2015). The Upside of Stress: Why Stress Is Good for You, and How to Get Good at It" *in Scientific American Mind* 26, 4, p. 70 (July 2015).

FDA. (2004). Suicidality in Children and Adolescents Being Treated With Antidepressant Medications **Available at:** https://www.fda.gov/drugs/postmarket-drug-safety-information-patients-and-providers/suicidality-children-and-adolescents-being-treated-antidepressant-medications#:~:text=Today%20the%20Food%20and%20Drug,and%20behavior)%20in%20children%20and (Accessed 27th February 2023).

Feder, A., Southwick, S. M., Goetz, R. R., Wang, Y., Alonso, A., Smith, B. W., Buchholz, K. R., Waldeck, T., Ameli, R., Moore, J., Hain, R., Charney, D. S. and Vythilingam, M. (2008) 'Posttraumatic growth in former Vietnam prisoners of war', *Psychiatry: Interpersonal & Biological Processes* 71 (4) pp. 359-370.

Flintham, A. (2003) *When reservoirs run dry: why some head-teachers leave headship early.* Nottingham, NCSL.

Forrest, L. (2008) 'The three faces of victim – an overview of the drama triangle', *lynneforrest. com.* Available at: www.lynneforrest.com/articles/2008/06/the-faces-of-victim/ (Accessed 26th July 2017).

Fotalia, L. (2017) 'The mere presence of your smartphone reduces brain power, study shows', *Science Daily.* Available at: www.sciencedaily.com/releases/2017/06/170623133039.htm (Accessed 24th August 2023).

Frozen (2013) Directed by Chris Buck [Film]. Burbank, CA: Walt Disney Studios Motion Pictures.

Gillie, O. (1977). "Did Sir Cyril Burt Fake His Research on Heritability of Intelligence? Part I". *The Phi Delta Kappan.* 58 (6): 469–71.

Gilligan, V. (2008 – 2013) Breaking Bad. Culver City, USA: Sony Pictures Television Inc.

Griffin, J. and Tyrrell, I. (2014a) *How to lift depression...fast.* Chalvington: Human Givens Publishing Ltd.

Griffin, J. and Tyrrell, I. (2014b) *Why we dream: the definitive answer.* Chalvington: Human Givens Publishing Ltd.

Goleman, D. (1998) *Working with emotional intelligence.* London: Bloomsbury.

Grossman, Paul; Taylor, Edwin W. (2007-02-01). Toward understanding respiratory sinus arrhythmia: Relations to cardiac vagal tone, evolution and biobehavioral functions". *Biological Psychology. 74 (2): 263–285.*

Harvey Practice (2022) *Message to Patients.* Merley: NHS.

Heinlein, R. (1953) *Assignment in Eternity* Pennsylvania; Fantasy Press.

Holloway, G (2023) Confessions of a Headmaster (1). San

Bruno, CA: You Tube. Available at https://www.youtube.com/watch?v=_YCql9FDt3M&t=72s. (Accessed 24th January 2023)

Hou, Y., Xiong, D., Jiang, T., Song, L., & Wang, Q. (2019). Social media addiction: Its impact, mediation, and intervention. Cyberpsychology: *Journal of Psychosocial Research on Cyberspace,* 13(1), article 4.

Irlenbusch, B. and Sliwka, D. (2005) *Incentives, Decision Frames, and Motivation Crowding Out – An Experimental Investigation.* Bonn: The Institute for the Study of Labor

Johnsen, T. J., & Friborg, O. (2015, May 11). The Effects of Cognitive Behavioral Therapy as an Anti-Depressive Treatment is Falling: A Meta-Analysis. *Psychological Bulletin.*

Junger, S. (1997) *The perfect storm: a true story of men against the sea.* Hammersmith: Harper.

Karpman, S. (1972) *Eric Berne memorial scientific award lecture.* Available at: www. karpmandramatriangle.com/pdf/AwardSpeech.pdf (Accessed 26th July 2017).

Keller, A., Litzelman, K., Wisk, L., Maddox, T., Cheng, E., Creswell, P. and Witt. W. (2012) *Does the Perception That Stress Affects Health Matter? The Association with Health and Mortality.* Wisconsin: Marquette University.

King, L. A., King, D. W., Fairbank, J. A., Keane, T. M. and Adams, G. A. (1998) 'Resilience- recovery factors in posttraumatic stress disorder among female and male Vietnam veterans: hardiness, postwar social support, and additional stressful life events', *Journal of Personality and Social Psychology* 74 (2) pp. 420–434.

Knight, S. Finlay, T. and Russell, S. (2013-2022) *Peaky Blinders.* London: BBC

Koestler, A. (1967). The Ghost in the Machine (1990 reprint ed.).

London: Penguin Group

Kubler – Ross, E. (1969) *On Death & Dying*. New York: Simon & Schuster.

Kumano, M (2018). "On the Concept of Well-Being in Japan: Feeling Shiawase as Hedonic Well-Being and Feeling Ikigai as Eudaimonic Well-Being". *Applied Research in Quality of Life*. 13 (2): 419–433.

Lancashire: NHS Foundation Trust Available at https://www.lscft.nhs.uk/media/Publications/Traumatic-Stress-Service/How-Trauma-Affects.pdf. (Accessed on 17th February 2022).

Levitin, D. J. (2015) 'Why the modern world is bad for your brain', *The Guardian*, 18th January. Available at: www.theguardian.com/science/2015/jan/18/modern-world-bad-for-brain-daniel-j-levitin-organized-mind-information-overload.

Liao, S. (2017) 'A five-minute meditation' in Gibbs, N. (ed.) *Mindfulness, a pathway to health and happiness*. New York, NY: Time Books.

Lord, C., Ross, L., & Lepper, M. (1979). Biased Assimilation and Attitude Polarization: The effects of Prior Theories on Subsequently Considered Evidence. *Journal of Personality and Social Psychology*, 37, 2098-2109.

Luders, E., Kurth, F., Mayer, E. A., Toga, A. W., Narr, K. L. and Gaser, C. (2012) 'The unique brain anatomy of meditation practitioners: alterations in cortical gyrification', *Frontiers in Human Neuroscience* 6 (34).

MacLean, Paul D. (1990). *The triune brain in evolution: role in paleocerebral functions*. New York: Plenum Press.

MacLean, P., (1990). *The triune brain in evolution: role in paleocerebral functions*. New York: Plenum Press.

Maggio, M., Colizzi, E., Fisichella, A., Valenti, G., Geresini, G., Dall'Aglioa, E., Ruffini, L., Lauretani, F., Parrino, L., Ceda,

G. (2013) *Stress hormones, sleep deprivation and cognition in older adults.* Amsterdam: Elsevier.

Maguire, E., Gadian, D., Johnsrude, J., Good, C., Ashburner, J., Frackowiak, R., and Frith, C. (2000) Navigation-related structural change in the hippocampi of Taxi Drivers. *Proceedings of the National Academy of Science of the United States of America.* 97(8):4398-403.

Maslow, A.(1943). A theory of human motivation. *Psychological Review.* 50 (4): 370–396.

Mary Poppins (1964). Burbank, Ca: Disney Motion Picture Studios.

McCann, I and Pearlman, L. (1960) Vicarious traumatization: A framework for understanding the psychological effects of working with victims. *Journal of Traumatic Stress,* 3(1), 131-149.

McGonical, K., (2015) *The Upside of Stress; why stress is good for you (and how to get good at it)* London: Vermillion.

McGonical, K. (2013) [TED talk] *How to make stress your friend.* Available at: https://www.youtube.com/watch?v=RcGyVTAoXEU (Accessed 5th February 2022).

Mercury, F. (1978) *Don't Stop Me Now.* London: Universal Publishing Group.

Mikulic, M (2023) *Pharmaceutical market: worldwide revenue 2001-2022.* Available at: https://www.statista.com/statistics/263102/pharmaceutical-market-worldwide-revenue-since-2001/#:~:text=For%202022%2C%20the%20total%20global,what%20people%20pay%20for%20medication. (Accessed 21st February 2023).

Milgram, Stanley (1967). "The Small World Problem". *Psychology Today.* 2: 60–67.

Miller, E. (2013) Digital *lives – the science behind*

multitasking [Video]. Available at: www.youtube. com/watch?v=E5JNpTySQ_8&t=13s (Accessed 10th March 2023) 2017).

Mortimer, B (2021) *And Away, the autobiography*. London: Gallery Books, UK

Moynihan R and Cassels A. (2005) *Selling Sickness: How Drug Companies are Turning Us All Into Patients*. NSW, Aus.: Allen and Unwin.

NHS (2017) 'Mindfulness', *NHS Choices*. Available at: www.nhs.uk/Conditions/stress-anxiety- depression/pages/mindfulness.aspx) (Accessed 1st September 2017).

National Institute for Health and Care Excellence (NICE) (2009). *Depression in adults: recognition and management* .Available at https://www.nice.org.uk/guidance/cg90/ifp/chapter/treatments-for-mild-to-moderate-depression (Accessed on 20/1/2022)

Naylor, L. (2022) Safeguarding. Beyond Education That Counts (Podcast) Available at https://linktr.ee/beyond_education. (Accessed on 24th April 2022).

Nelms, J., & Castel, D. (2016). A Systematic Review and Meta-Analysis of Randomized and Non-Randomized Trials of Emotional Freedom Techniques (EFT) for the Treatment of Depression. Explore: The Journal of Science and Healing, 12, 416-426.

Nursing Times (2013) Controversy over DSM-5: new mental health guide. Available at: https://www.nursingtimes.net/news/behind-the-headlines/controversy-over-dsm-5-new-mental-health-guide-24-08-2013/ (Accessed 22nd February 2023).

Ochsner, K. N., Ray, R. D., Cooper, J. C., Robertson, E. R., Chopra, S., Gabrieli, J. D. and Gross, J. J. (2004). 'For better or for worse: neural systems supporting the cognitive down- and up-regulation of negative emotion', *Neuroimage* 23 (2) pp. 483-499.

Peck, S. (1978) *The Road Less Travelled*. London: Ebury Press.

Pérez-Carbonell, L, Meurling, I, Wassermann, D, Gnoni, I, Leschziner, G, Weighall, A, Ellis, J, Durrant, S, Hare, A and Steier, J1 (2020) Impact of the novel coronavirus (COVID-19) pandemic on sleep *Journal of Thoracic Disease* Vol 12, Supplement 2 (October 15, 2020):

Pickersgill, M. (2013) *Debating DSM-5, diagnosis and the sociology of critique*. London, BMJ journals.

Pink, D. (2009) *Drive: The Surprising Truth About What Motivates Us*. New York: Penguin Books (USA inc).

Porges SW (2011). *The Polyvagal Theory: Neurophysiological Foundations of Emotions, Attachment, Communication, and Self-regulation*. New York: WW Norton.

Raiders of the Lost Ark (1981) Directed by Steven Spielberg (Film). Hollywood, CA: Paramount.

Ramachandran, V.S. (2012) *The tell-tale brain: a neuroscientist's quest for what makes us human*. London: Windmill Books.

Ricard, M. (2025). *Altruism. The Science and Psychology of Kindness*. London: Atlantic Books

Robinson, J (2021) NHS spending on antidepressants rose by £139m during pandemic, study finds. Available at : https://pharmaceutical-journal.com/article/news/nhs-spending-on-antidepressants-rose-by-139m-during-pandemic-study-finds (Accessed 27th February 2023).

Robotham, D., Chakkalackal, L. and Cyhlarova, E. (2011) *The impact of sleep on health and wellbeing*. London: Mental Health Foundation.

Rottenberg, J. (2014) *The depths: the evolutionary origins of the depression epidemic*. New York NY: Basic Books.

Rittel, H. W. J. and Webber, M. M. (1973) 'Dilemmas in a general theory of planning', *Policy Sciences* 4 (2) pp. 155-169.

Sagan, C. (1977) (1977). The Dragons of Eden: Speculations on the Evolution of Human Intelligence (1st ed.). New York: Random House.

Santamauro, D. (2021) Global prevalence and burden of depressive and anxiety disorders in 204 countries and territories in 2020 due to the COVID-19 pandemic. *The Lancet 2021*; 398: 1700–12 Available at https://doi.org/10.1016/ S0140-6736(21)02143-7 (Accessed 20/1/2022).

Savage, A. (2006) *Slow leadership: civilising the organization.* Australia: Pusch Ridge Publishing.

Scott, M (2022) *The Facebook whistleblower takes on the metaverse.* Washington; Politico.

Sebastian B, Nelms J. The Effectiveness of Emotional Freedom Techniques in the Treatment of Post Traumatic Stress Disorder: A Meta-Analysis. *Explore*: New York. 2017 Jan-Feb;13(1):16-25.

Seligman, M. (1988) 'People born after 1945 were ten times more likely to suffer from depression than people born 50 years earlier' in Buie, J. (ed.) *'Me' decades generate depression: individualism erodes commitment to others.* Washington, DC: APA Monitor.

Seligman, M. (1972) 'Learned helplessness', *Annual Review of Medicine* 23 (1) pp. 407-412.

Seligman, M. E. P., & Csikszentmihalyi, M. (2000). Positive psychology: An introduction. *American Psychologist, 55*(1), pp. 5–14.

Seligman, M. 2002). *Authentic Happiness: Using the New Positive Psychology to Realize Your Potential for Lasting Fulfilment.* . New York: Free Press.

Seligman, M. (2008) *The new era of positive psychology* [TED Talk]. Available at: www.youtube. com/watch?v=9FBxfd7DL3E (Accessed 21st February 2023).

Selye, H, (1956) *The Stress of Life*. New York: McGraw-Hill.

Sills, J. (2013) 'The power of no', *Psychology today*. Available at: www.psychologytoday.com/ articles/201311/the-power-no (Accessed 20th July 2023).

Sleepio (2011) *The Great British sleep survey: new data on the impact of poor sleep*. Available at: www.greatbritishsleepsurvey.com/ (Accessed 27th January 2023).

Sleepio (2012) *The Great British sleep survey: new data on the impact of poor sleep*. Available at: www.greatbritishsleepsurvey.com/ (Accessed 27th January 2023).

Solms, M. (2000) 'Dreaming and REM sleep are controlled by different brain mechanisms', *Behavioral and Brain Sciences* 23 (6) pp. 843-850.

Southwick and Charney (2013) 'Ready for anything', *Scientific American Mind* 24 (3) pp. 32-41.

Stapleton, P (2022) *Overview Document, Energy Psychology and EFT/Tapping*. Available at: https://s3.amazonaws.com/kajabi-storefronts-production/file-uploads/sites/2147597324/themes/2151516842/downloads/e145dba-d04-8f50-ffa7-7c7f5c6ced5_EBEFT_Overview_of_Research_2022.pdf (Accessed 28th February 2023)

Steele, C & Aronson, J (1995) *Stereotype Threat and Intellectual Test Performance of African Americans*, Journal of Personality and Social Psychology Vo. 69 No.5.

Sternlicht, L. and Sternlicht, A. (2023) A New Age of Digital Addiction - What The Metaverse Means for Mental Health and Digital Addiction. Available at: https://www.family-addictionspecialist.com/blog/a-new-age-of-digital-addiction-what-the-metaverse-means-for-mental-health-and-digital-addiction#:~:text=The%20Metaverse%20and%20Mental%20Health,%2C%20and%20psychoses%2C%20among%20others. (Accessed 29th August 2023)

Swan, P (2009). *Diary of a Bomb Aimer and Training in America and Flying with 12 Squadron in WW ll.* Barnsley: Pen and Sword Aviation.

Sweller, J (1988). "Cognitive load during problem solving: Effects on learning". *Cognitive Science.* 12 (2): 257–285.

Tawakol, A., Ishai, I., Takx, R., Figuero, A., Adelrahman, A., Kaiser, Y., Truong, Q., Solomon, C., Calcagno, C., Mani, V., Tang, C., Mulder, W., Morrough, J., Hoffmann, U., Nahrendorf, M., Shin, L., Fayad, Z. Pitman, R (2017) Relation between resting amygdalar activity and cardiovascular events: a longitudinal and cohort study. Lancet. 2017 Feb 25; 389(10071) pp. 834–845.

The Guardian (2017) 'The *Guardian* view on betting terminals: an outrageous racket', 20th August. Available at: www.theguardian.com/commentisfree/2017/aug/20/the-guardian-view-on-betting-terminals-an-outrageous-racket

The Lancet (2003) *How a Statin Might Destroy a Drug Company.* Available at: https://www.thelancet.com/journals/lancet/article/PIIS0140-6736(03)12723-7/fulltext (Accessed 2nd February 2023).

The Priory (2021) Available at: https://www.priorygroup.com/mental-health/mental-health-statistics. (Accesed 17th March 2023)

The Revenant (2015) Directed by Alejandro G. Inarritu [Film]. Los Angeles, CA: 20th Century Fox.

Thomas, W. (2016) Soul Candy. Stroud: Chrysalis Poetry.

Toffler, A. (1970) Future Shock. London: The Bodley Head.

Torjesen, I (2020) Covid-19: Mental health services must be boosted to deal with "tsunami" of cases after lockdown. BMJ 2020;369:m1994.

Tyrrell, M. (2007) *Emotional trance states*. Oban: Uncommon Knowledge.

Tyrrell, M. (2015) *Uncommon Psychotherapy. Oban:* Uncommon Knowledge Ltd.

University of Stanford (2021) GSBGEN 622: Presentation and Communication Skills for Academics. Available at: https://explorecourses.stanford.edu/search?q=GSBGEN%20622&academicYear=20202021 (Accessed 13th February 2022).

U.S. Department of Veteran Affairs. (2012). *VHA Handbook 1160.04, VHA Programs for Veterans with Substance Use Disorders (SUD).* Retrieved from: http://www.va.gov/vhapublications/publications.cfm?pub=2&order=asc&orderby=pub_Number (Accessed 27th April 2022).

Verderese, M. and H. *Roth (2011). "Kekulé's Dream"* Available at: https://web.*chemdoodle*.com/*kekules-dream/* (Accessed 5th May 2023)

Walker, R., (2019) Stressed Brits buy record number of self-help books The Guardian. 9th March 2019. Available at: https://www.theguardian.com/books/2019/mar/09/self-help-books-sstressed-brits-buy-record-number (Accessed 9th February 2020).

Ward, A., Duke, K., Gneezy, A. and Bos, M. (2017) 'Brain drain: the mere presence of one's own smartphone reduces available cognitive capacity', *Journal of the Association for Consumer Research* 2 (2) pp. 140-154.

Weil, A. (2015) *Asleep in 60 seconds* [Video]. Available at: www.youtube.com/watch?v=gz4G31LGyog (Accessed 30th August 2017).

Wells, M. (2014), *Courage and Air Warfare: The Allied Aircrew Experience in the Second World War*, Routledge.

Westen, D., Blagov, S., Harenski, K., Kilts, C. and Hamann, S. (2006) 'Neural bases of motivated reasoning: an FMRI study of emotional constraints on partisan political judgment in the 2004 US presidential election', *Journal of Cognitive Neuroscience* 18 (11) pp. 1947-1958.

Wiliam, D. (1998). Enculturating learners into communities of practice: raising achievement through classroom practice. Available at: https://scholar.google.co.uk/scholar?q=dylan+wiliam+ego+and+task+feedback+pdf&hl=en&as_sdt=0&as_vis=1&oi=scholart (Accessed 27th July 2023).

Williams, A. and Head, V. (2006). *Terror Attacks: The Violent Expression of Desperation – Attack on the Royal Marine School of Music*. London: Futura.

Wong, Y., Owen, J., Gabana, N., Brown, J. McInnis, S., Toth, P. and Gilman, L. (2018) Does gratitude writing improve the mental health of psychotherapy clients? Evidence from a randomized controlled trial. Psychotherapy Research. 2018 Mar;28(2):192-202.

World Health Organisation (2021) *Depression* Available at: https://www.who.int/news-room/fact-sheets/detail/depression (Accessed 21st February 2023).

Zimmerman, C., Leib, D. and Knight, Z (2017) Neural circuits underlying thirst and fluid homeostasis. *Nature Reviews Neuroscience* 18, pp 459–469.

Milton Keynes UK
Ingram Content Group UK Ltd.
UKHW030955120824
446802UK00011B/212